Celebrate Life

New Attitudes for Living
with Chronic Illness

KATHLEEN LEWIS

D0965419

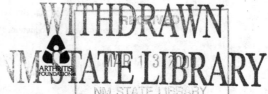

PUBLISHED BY
THE ARTHRITIS FOUNDATION

Published by
Arthritis Foundation
1330 West Peachtree Street
Atlanta, GA 30309

Library of Congress Catalog Card Number 99-65981
ISBN: 0-912423-24-2

Printed in the United States of America

Editorial Director: ELIZABETH AXTELL
Art Director: AUDREY GRAHAM

Manuscript Editor: Krista Reese
Illustration: Kat Thacker
Interior layout & production: Jill Dible

*What the caterpillar thinks is the end,
the butterfly knows is just the beginning.*

Dedication

Celebrate Life: New Attitudes for Living With Chronic Illness began in March 1981 as a column called "Let's Celebrate Life" in a newsletter, *Horizons*, published by the Greater Atlanta Chapter of the Lupus Foundation. Two previous renditions of this book were published under the title *Successful Living With Chronic Illness: Celebrating the Joys of Life.*

Each chapter began with the blood, sweat and tears of my life and experience. Each page contains a part of my struggles, defeats and victories.

I hope that whatever I share of my story will help at least one person in his or her journey with chronic illness.

This book is designed for people with chronic illness and their doctors, families and friends. And though I hope that many others will find the information given here useful, I'd like our conversation as writer and reader to be as intimate as possible. For that reason, I will be directly addressing you, the reader who is struggling with illness.

I dedicate *Celebrate Life* to you, the readers who breathed life into this book by making it a part of your lives. You have made this updated edition possible.

Table of Contents

Foreword ix
Acknowledgements xi
My Story xiii

PART III Learning the Medical Ropes

PART IV Making Changes

PART V Celebrating Life

Foreword

Years ago, I received an unsolicited manuscript concerning living with chronic illness, which its author asked me, in my role as editor-in-chief of *Postgraduate Medicine*, to consider for publication. The subject is an important one for the doctors our journal serves – family physicians, general internists and other primary care physicians – but, frankly, not a very exciting one. The submitted manuscript did little to spark my interest. It was dull and pedantic, filled with psychobabble.

I returned the essay to the author with a candid opinion, pointing out the rather stilted language and stating my belief that our readers simply would not read this. Having rejected the article, I quickly put it out of my mind. Therefore, I was somewhat surprised to receive a revised manuscript a few weeks later.

"Revised" is an inadequate term, however, to describe this new manuscript, which bore little or no resemblance to the earlier version. I was now reading a compassionate, personal and moving account of living with chronic illness – the ups and downs, the sadness and grief, the changes in lifestyle and in personal relationships that occur when one is so afflicted. I promptly accepted the article, and it was published under the title "Living with Chronic Illness: Dying is the Easy Part," in our September 1983 issue.

This experience constituted my introduction to Kathleen S. Lewis. Subsequently, through continuing correspondence, I have come to know her as an unusually gifted person, a person with special perception and inspired insights she shares with us here. Her intelligence, her strength of will and her intense religious faith are all evident throughout.

Ms. Lewis' work deserves to be read by physicians, who will be immensely helped in their understanding of what their chronically ill patients are going through. It should be read by friends and relatives of such patients, people who are so essential in constituting the support group for the sick person. These people will find out how important their roles are and learn much about how they may best fulfill them.

Most importantly, of course, the book should be read by every patient suffering from a chronic disease. It is a rich compendium of philosophical advice that concerns dealing with and ultimately accepting one's infirmity, as well as a group of helpful pragmatic hints about dealing with specific situations, such as visiting one's doctor. We should be grateful to Ms. Lewis for shedding new light on this shadowed area.

Robert B. Howard, MD

Acknowledgments

My thanks to the Arthritis Foundation and the Atlanta chapter of the Lupus Foundation of America for recognizing the value of my work to those who struggle daily with chronic illness. The benefit of the patient has remained the underlying motivation of all involved.

Special thanks to the following individuals who reviewed this book and shared their insightful comments: Stephen T. Wegener, PhD; Saralynn H. Allaire, RNScD; and Kathleen M. Schiaffino, PhD.

My Story

I was born December 4, 1944, on a farm in Greenville, S.C. The delivery was difficult for my 39-year-old mother: I came out feet first, with the umbilical cord around my neck. Mother had been hospitalized for several weeks for complications in the pregnancy. But despite warnings about her health, she and my father, then 47, had decided that after adopting two boys, they desperately wanted another child.

On our 30-acre farm, we grew cotton, corn and wheat, and raised horses, cows, chickens and pigs. I raised and trained my own mare. I remember sowing seeds in the pasture with my father, who would scatter huge handfuls for large distances as I'd dribble a few grains here and there along the way.

I became a tomboy, fighting my brothers to let me play on the football or baseball team in the pasture. I rode my horse bareback and without a bridle. Mother would sign me up for typing and home economics classes in school. I would change them to biology and chemistry. My grandmother, Mother Reaves, would try to bribe me to learn to cook and sew. I'd slip out to the ball field, barn or lake.

My father was always busy on the farm (he was out killing hogs when I was born) when he wasn't selling insurance or involved in political interests. Mother was a talented amateur artist, painting oils, pastels and watercolors of all kinds, from still life to portraits. Sometimes she would sell a few of her works.

Our maid, Tex Anna Jones, came to the family when I was a year old. She became my spiritual and emotional mother, demonstrating feeling in a way our family never had. Anna taught me how to *celebrate life* as she stood on a chair and screamed at a mouse, hid in the hall closet during a thunderstorm, hummed gospel songs as she ironed, or simply, freely and deeply laughed.

From an early age, I connected with nature and pondered its creator. Rainbows, sunsets, storm clouds, butterflies – all seemed full of spirit and meaning. Even when I was very young, I was active in our Southern Baptist church with choir, missions and youth activities. As I grew older, I felt the call to become a missionary nurse. I applied for and was accepted to Vanderbilt University School of Nursing in Nashville, Tenn., where I eventually earned my nursing degree.

Before I headed off to school, my mother and grandmother sat me down and let me in on a carefully guarded family secret. My mother had struggled most of her life with manic depression (now called bipolar disorder). I was shocked – as I was growing up, I knew only that there were times when Mother would suddenly paint five paintings a week, and other times when she couldn't seem to function very well.

The fact that Mother Reaves always either lived next to us or with us began to make more sense; I finally understood why we needed a maid. The family had kept my mother's problem hidden because they were ashamed of the stigma of mental illness. I didn't understand until later that as my mother and grandmother told me her secret, they were preparing me for the role of her emotional caretaker.

After only a couple of weeks away at Vanderbilt, I fell hard for a red-headed, energetic premed student. Like me, Jim Lewis also felt the call to missions. At the end of our freshman year, with fear in his heart that he would lose me, he told me that he felt he wanted to be a preacher rather than a doctor. Time reaffirmed my love for him, and we began to plan a life together.

In summers between academic years, I sought challenging work. I found it in places like Greenville's Shriners Crippled Children's Hospital and the charity ward at Greenville General Hospital, where sick or injured prisoners were sent. That summer, I learned some words I hadn't known existed.

Jim and I were married January 29, 1966. In the fall, we headed off to Southern Baptist Theological Seminary in Louisville, Ky. For the next eight years, as Jim earned his doctorate, I worked as a nurse to help support us. While studying, Jim served as pastor at Northfork Baptist Church for six years in Frankfort, Ky., where our two sons, Jamie and Keith, were born, in 1968 and 1970.

Mother Reaves had died while I was in college. My father died of a heart attack in 1971. After Anna died a year later, my mother's emotional care fell to me. We still lived far apart, but I kept in close touch with her by phone. She was able to stay in the colonial mansion she and Daddy had built, but Mother relied heavily on Jim and me for emotional support and decisions. Lithium seemed to level off her highs and lows, and in her better times, she even enjoyed traveling abroad. She no longer painted copiously.

Much to my surprise, over the years I realized that no one else in the family knew Mother's secret. My brothers, uncle and aunt seemed quite surprised when I would mention Mother's difficulties. Later, after I became ill, when her condition required regular hospitalization in a psychiatric ward, they simply couldn't – or wouldn't – believe what I was telling them.

For my husband and me, it was a time of growth in our

careers in nursing and ministry, even with the demands of our extended family. After seminary, we moved to Baltimore, Md., to serve as language missionaries for the Home Mission Board of the Southern Baptist Convention. Our job was to reach out to the many foreign-language churches and congregations in the northeast. I also worked as a visiting nurse in the inner city. After Jim joined the Home Mission Board staff, we moved to Atlanta, Ga., where I again joined the ranks of visiting nurses working in the inner city.

My life was crammed with activity. Still trim and athletic, I loved nothing more than being outdoors. Besides raising my two sons, trying to be a good wife, emotionally supporting my mother and working full-time in a stressful job, I wedged in hobbies and other pastimes. I was as active as ever in my church and loved singing in the choir.

However, I'd also been nagged by mysterious health problems for years, starting with painful joints and frequent infections. Most of the time, I ignored my symptoms and pushed on with my busy life. My condition would fluctuate between good and bad. In 1978, I was diagnosed with systemic lupus erythematosus (SLE). It was the first of several serious diagnoses.

My life blew up in my face. My healthy, tanned body grew pale, blotchy and weak. I was forced to give up so many of the things I loved to do. My nursing career evaporated and I went on disability. My family, so dependent on me, waited for me to get well. I didn't.

I read the little I could get my hands on about emotional and physical adjustment to a chronic illness. I learned how people's psychological problems could be more crippling and long-lasting than their physical ailments. I began to observe how people's emotional reactions to chronic illness made all the difference in whether they were able to go on with life.

Though I'd never written before in my life, I found that putting my thoughts on paper helped clear my clouded mind. I kept a prayer journal. Letters became a valuable connection with the world. Poems began to pour out of me. Eventually, I began writing articles on a wide variety of topics.

In time, after publishing some of my pieces, I had the audacity to begin calling myself a freelance writer. In 1985, I published a book, *Successful Living With Chronic Illness: Celebrating the Joys of Life*, which had evolved from a newsletter column. Radio and TV interviews and invitations to speak around the country followed.

I slowly began to realize that my life, as I'd known it, was over. In order to let go of that past life so that I could begin another, I needed to grieve my losses. Grieving can make you feel very alone – few are able to stand by you through that long, difficult process. My own often lonely experience with grief led me to seek out and voluntarily counsel people who had suffered a loss. Week after week, people who had lost a job, a spouse or a child came to talk about whatever they needed to talk about. I listened and learned.

At about that time, a local Baptist hospital with a chaplaincy training program offered ministers' wives an introductory experience as hospital chaplains. I accepted, although my diminished health meant I was barely able to make it through the scheduled group supervision sessions and patient visits two mornings a week. The program stretched into nine months, during which an SLE flare landed me in bed for three months and the hospital for a week. I was able to return and finish the program later.

After this chaplaincy experience, I wondered if I might be able to offer counseling after a loss, which I called grief support, in a professional capacity. I enrolled in Georgia State University's master's degree program in rehabilitation counseling, which seemed to address the physical and emotional struggle of coming to terms with illness or disability. I took the program one test, one paper, one course, one quarter at a time, without ever expecting to finish. From time to time I needed to drop out. Rather than give me an incomplete, my professors would give me an "in progress."

With my professors' permission, I geared each course to chronic illness, writing every paper and designing every project to address the subject. The faculty was understanding as I landed in the hospital, underwent six surgeries, studied, wrote and counseled over the phone from my bed or the hospital many times. Incredibly, I won a literary award that usually went to doctoral-level candidates. Many professors would comment that I knew more about the emotional aspects of chronic illness than they did.

Meanwhile, I'd discovered that lupus had given me a mandate to become healthier emotionally and spiritually – which in turn helped balance my physical state. I was learning how to ask for what I needed and to set boundaries without getting sick. Before I became ill, I didn't know I had boundaries or that I needed anything, much less what. Slowly over many years, my illness became just a part of me and not all of me. A different person was emerging from my grief cocoon, and I liked her.

Along the path to emotional health, I learned a lot about myself. In growing up, I'd adopted the role of caretaker in my relationships, and my illness forced me to resign from that job. Those changes meant I couldn't continue to be responsible for the emotional well-being of my mother, who began to require hospitalization after I was diagnosed. My shifts also upset the balance and fit of my marriage.

Under the stresses of our family life, job, school and my illness, and struggling with his own midlife crisis, Jim left our marriage in 1984. We divorced two heartache-filled years later. I am seeing that pain and sorrow redeemed now as I counsel, write and speak about chronic illness and the family.

I completed my master's in rehabilitation counseling in 1986. It had taken me five years, a pace my body could withstand, to finish a program that usually took a year and a half. I later began a counseling ministry in my home.

Getting into family counseling with my sons helped me to stay sane. In Family and Marriage Counseling courses at the University of Georgia, I wrote papers based on a genogram from my own family. A genogram traces the emotional patterns in three generations. Wow! Was that ever difficult, painful work!

I believe my emotional inheritance helped trigger my illness. I was raised as a codependent caretaker. Codependent people end up enabling unhealthy behavior in others, just as partners of alcoholics sometimes unconsciously make it possible for the alcoholic to continue drinking by making excuses for him, giving him money or rationalizing his behavior. I had unconsciously colluded with my mother's and husband's dependence on me by swooping in to emotionally rescue them. It was a pattern I would repeat in every relationship and setting in which I was involved.

I was trying so hard to take care of the world that I hadn't taken care of myself. Somehow, I could be my own caretaker only when I was ill. A genetic predisposition "wired" me for lupus, but stress and overwork – partly from codependent relationships – may have helped trigger it.

Obviously, it's impossible to turn back the clock. But becoming conscious of my motives and actions allows me to make healthy choices rather than repeating unhealthy, unconscious reactive patterns. In some families, these patterns continue unbroken for generations.

Today, I still counsel families on a volunteer basis, at home and through my church's divorce recovery support group. I've also been involved in the Arthritis Foundation's SLE Self-Help (SLESH) course since 1981. I went to Arizona for my first SLESH training in 1984, just after my husband had left me. Plastering a smile on my face, I'd go to classes, only to return to my room and dissolve into tears. One part of my life was dying, and I was undergoing another difficult birth.

Every ending is truly a new beginning.

On my business card as a counselor, I adopted the butterfly as a personal logo. Lupus often leaves its mark in the form of a butterfly-shaped facial rash. The butterfly also represents the death of one form of life and the beginning of a beautiful new one.

I'm continually thrust into new directions, learning about myself, others and the spirit that binds us all. I've found a mission field, but not the one I expected: It's among those whose lives have been touched by illness and divorce and who, in turn, touch my life. I can only hope to emulate my father's capacity for sowing a large swath of seeds instead of just dribbling a few seeds here and there.

Before the end of my mother's life, we were able to establish a healthier, more balanced relationship. I'd respond to her anxious calls by telling her I wasn't going to worry about her problems because I knew she would and could take care of them. She began to assume responsibility for herself. In her later years, she began a long and slow physical decline that started with a broken hip. Her last eight years in a nursing home were extremely hard for both of us.

My two sons are now grown up, and both work in the food industry. Keith is a chef and is married to a chef. Jamie supervises several pizza stores. I am often amazed at all they have experienced in their young lives. I am proud to be their mom.

My own life lessons are shared in this book. Not all of them are academic. Though I've spent a good deal of time in the classroom, I have learned more about chronic illness as a patient than I ever did as a professional. Lessons on paper have become a living reality, defined by unforgettable personal experience. It's a school I'll never graduate from, nor carry any degrees or titles except that of fellow struggler or wounded healer.

Since the first edition of this book, I've begun dating again, have gone through menopause, and have gone whitewater rafting and hang gliding. My license plate reads JOY-AWE. I am overjoyed and awed to be alive, sane and happy! I have been through the depths of the valleys and soared above mountaintops. In my journey with chronic illness, I've discovered that:

There can be victory in defeat,
gain in loss,
living in dying,
wholeness in brokenness,
giving in receiving,
success in failure,
strength in weakness,

peace in turmoil,
joy in sorrow,
growth in pain, and
mental health in the midst of physical illness!

This book isn't mine to crow about. It belongs to you, the reader, and where you are on your journey through life. Nothing I say is grand, wonderful, exciting or profound unless it connects with you. If anything here helps you make it one step or minute further in your life, we've shared a victory. Bon voyage!

PART I

Integrating the Illness
Into Your Life

CHAPTER 1

How Do You Spell Relief?
D-I-A-G-N-O-S-I-S

The Diagnostic Crazies: A Play in Many Acts

The Dialogue

"Listen, Doc, what's going on? I have all these aches and pains. I feel lousy all the time. I'm tired, grouchy and just can't seem to function like I used to. I push and try, but I just can't get my act together."

"I feel so angry and guilty. My husband, family and friends can't understand why I'm acting so strangely. Neither can I. Friends are getting tired of asking how I'm doing. When they ask what's wrong, I don't know what to tell them anymore.

"My boss thinks I'm dragging my feet and has made hints about his dissatisfaction with my performance. I should be in line for a promotion and raise about now, but instead, I'm afraid he may fire me if I don't straighten up and get back to 'normal.' I feel like I'm getting to be a chronic complainer and

I was never that way before now. I used to be such a positive, active person. I feel like I'm becoming a different person!

"I don't know how much longer all these people are going to have patience with me without some answers as to what's going on. Please tell me what's wrong with me so I can take some medicine and get on with my life! You've run so many tests. I don't want anything to be wrong with me, but I know there has to be or I wouldn't be feeling as bad as I do. Please, tell me what I have ... now!!"

The Setting

Sitting in the same room, facing this distraught person (maybe you), is a physician who has devoted his or her life to a career in medicine, sometimes at great financial and personal sacrifice. He uses all his knowledge and experience to put the pieces of the puzzle together and come up with a correct diagnosis.

In response to your insistent, impassioned pleas, the physician may be tempted to hastily put a diagnosis on your chart, just to have the matter settled and get you out of his hair. It takes much greater honesty to say, "No, I don't know exactly what is going on with you."

Your doctor may also be reluctant to jump to a conclusion of a chronic illness, because having that label on your chart could lead to discrimination by insurance companies and employers. Your doctor may be trying to protect you by holding out on the definitive diagnosis until he or she is absolutely sure.

The Characters

You have your own beliefs, attitudes and conceptions about illness, together with all kinds of good and bad prejudices about doctors. Some of these ideas may be generated from the myth concerning the power of our modern technology and medicine and the perception of the physician as god-like.

You may be sitting there thinking that any condition can be easily diagnosed, or that there is a cure or pill for your every ache and pain. Why, you know it's so, because you've seen it on TV! Rather than thinking of medicine as an imperfect, fallible science, you may view it as a perfect, infallible science. *It isn't.*

On the other hand, the physician may be sitting there, knowing that medicine has many limitations, even when at its best. Many conditions, such as neuromuscular abnormalities, connective tissue or immune system illnesses, can be very difficult to diagnose. Diagnosing them may require time, meticulous lab work-ups, thorough medical histories, and sometimes trials on medication. Even with the diagnosis, there may be no cure or treatment with easy answers, but only trial-and-error to see what helps.

Here you have two people approaching diagnosis from two different viewpoints – one very personal, and one professional as well as personal. You may be so frustrated you're bordering on becoming irrational, with diagnosis becoming an obsession.

You both want answers. But more than likely, when the answers and diagnosis you have been waiting for arrive, they aren't what you wanted to hear. At first, you may be greatly relieved to finally have a diagnosis. Up to that point, you may have felt your whole being and credibility were on the line. Am I sick, or am I crazy?

The physician is probably there for many reasons – to make a living, to practice his learned profession, to help people. He wants to be correct in his diagnosis and may be just as frustrated as you are, for different reasons. He or she must maintain some professional cool so that the situation can be viewed with clinical objectivity. To some degree, the physician's credibility may also be on the line.

After the Show
Post-Diagnosis

For the physician, a correct diagnosis may represent a validation of his professional expertise and positive strokes for his ego, as well as the personal gratification of helping another human being. Though symptoms can be treated before a diagnosis is rendered, sometimes the diagnosis marks a starting point for a whole philosophy of treatment and monitoring of the disease. But with many chronic illnesses, the doctor is limited to treating symptoms rather than the disease itself.

Some doctors may be more adept at diagnosis, while others may be better attuned to treatment. In fact, reaching a diagnosis may not change the treatment of your symptoms at all.

A number of changes occur as you are diagnosed. You now take on a new identity.

By this point, you may have had serious doubts about yourself and your sanity. Family, friends or physicians may even have expressed doubts about your mental health along the way. When the experiences of the outside world and your inner world don't correlate, you have a unique type of insanity. But now, with diagnosis, your internal experience, being sick, is verified externally. You may feel at last a meshing of inner and external experience. Then again, your worst fears may be realized, putting you to yet another test.

Result One: With a diagnosis, your perceptions of your inner reality are validated in your external world. You may experience a honeymoon period of relief before beginning to adjust. The diagnosis that you feared and may not be quite ready to accept is validated. It has been put into words, and typed in bold print on both your chart and your life.

Result Two: Diagnosis can dispel some unknowns and create others. With or without a diagnosis, you will be anxious and fearful about the unknowns and uncertainties in your life. But there may not be answers to every question.

Putting a diagnosis of a disease on an illness does, at least, condense what you are experiencing into a more manageable form of communication. A single word or grouping of words can replace the long list of complaints used previously to explain what is wrong with you. Your own subjective experience may be questioned, but an objective label given by a physician is an undeniable, authentic description that most people don't question.

A diagnosis of a recognized disease is essential when trying to communicate your needs officially to, for example, employers, insurance companies or disability reviews. Vague complaints and symptoms just don't cut it in this arena.

At the same time, a diagnosis can become a label that allows people to put you in a box. They can't see beyond that label to get to know you. A diagnosis of a medically and publicly recognized disease can confine as well as liberate you.

Result Three: A diagnosis can be a useful communication tool in many situations, but it can also be used by others to confine you to that label, never bothering to get to know the rest of you.

An official diagnostic decree uttered by a physician puts what you are experiencing into definite descriptive terms. This decree allows you to feel bad, to own what you are experiencing as illness. It thereby gives you permission and a mandate to take care of yourself and not try so hard to appear "normal."

You can now give in to your fatigue or pain and do something about it, rather than bravely push on. At the same time, you may need to sit down and take a long, hard look at the way you are going about your life, making some drastic, unwanted changes in lifestyle.

Result Four: A diagnosis may give you permission to take care of yourself, but it may also be a mandate that brings about many unwelcome changes in the way you live and how you view yourself.

Your dream of diagnosis, treatment, relief of symptoms and an improved lifestyle may only partially come true. For some, diagnosis becomes more than a dream – it becomes the pot of gold at the end of the rainbow, the proof that you were right, the answer to all your questions and the solution to all problems.

As with the doctor, the diagnosis only serves as a sober beginning, not the end of a quest. Some problems aren't going to go away and may need to be lived with, and more problems than solutions may be created.

A diagnosis can be a short-lived victory but it can give guidance and clarification to what has been happening to you. It is much easier to live with some unknowns than with all unknowns.

Result Five: A diagnosis is just the beginning of a journey. It opens the door to perhaps a few new problems, but may close the door on some old ones.

Moving On

Many times in my own journey with chronic illness, I might have sold my soul for a diagnosis ... the diagnostic crazies! I had desperately needed the relief of answers to the "whys" of my body's limitations.

I'd sometimes enter a bargaining mode, questioning everyone and asking for every conceivable diagnostic test because I couldn't just trust my internal reality. I'd make a diagnosis my main focus, thinking it would bring some relief.

Sometimes, after many years there would be an additional diagnosis – fibromyalgia, Sjögrens, Raynauds, osteoarthritis, carpal tunnel, exertional asthma. Sometimes there'd be no new label to explain what was happening to me.

I learned to try to trust myself and what my body was telling me about my limitations, take charge of my life and self, and not make a diagnosis my main goal in life. Diagnosis or not, I needed to grieve my lost functions and capacities knowing that the relief from a diagnosis is only for a brief period of time.

You need to develop a partnership with your doctor. For the partnership to happen, you, the patient, need to assume responsibility for yourself on a mind, body and spirit level ... the beginning of health.

You need to become the expert or specialist on you and your health and illness. Everybody is different and responds to illness differently. Become acquainted with your individual responses and communicate that to your doctor.

CHAPTER 2

Grief and Chronic Illness

The Stages of Grief

Your emotional reaction to a chronic illness can be determined by several factors.

1. Personality before the illness.
2. Unresolved grief or anger from the past.
3. The suddenness, extent and duration of lifestyle changes mandated by the illness.
4. Familial and individual resources for dealing with stress.
5. Stage of development of the individual and the family.
6. Previous experience with illness or crisis.
7. Codependcy within the family system.

Grief is seen as natural and even expected in the loss of a loved one. How much more intense and magnified grief may become when the loved one you're mourning is you!

Your losses from chronic illness are not, of course, as obvious as death. But you'll need to mourn your lost health, abilities and expectations, so that you can pick up the threads of your new life ... as it is now.

Loss and change are normal parts of life and aging. Chronic illness accelerates losses, and makes them undeniable.

A great deal has been written about the grief involved in facing terminal illness. Very little has been written about grief in chronic illness. Some even question the need to greive with a chronic illness. There are many comparisons and some distinctions between the two situations. With chronic and terminal illness, you may experience grief in reaction to the small losses along the way. You also may encounter that ultimate loss in death or shortened life span with both types of illness. In chronic illness, your losses are spread out over a lifetime.

Dr. Elisabeth Kübler-Ross's famous work, *On Death and Dying*, lists the stages of grief in terminal illness as denial, anger, bargaining, depression and acceptance.

For many people with chronic illnesses, you can add relief as the first stage, after finally getting a diagnosis. Very often, years may pass between the onset of symptoms and a doctor's decree. In my case, eight years of quirky health problems went by before I was diagnosed. A brief honeymoon period of relief followed.

After rejoicing in finally getting answers to the "come-and-go weirditis," I became scared to death I was going to die. I wrote letters for my family to find in the event of my death. Over the weeks, months, years, I began to realize I was going to live, but many aspects of the old Kathleen Lewis were lost. I needed to grieve those losses.

Each stage of grief has its benefits and dangers. You remain healthy only as you stay balanced and cycle in and out of the stages over a lifetime. If you get stuck in any one stage, you become unhealthy in your emotional approach to handling the illness.

Kübler-Ross distinguishes between reactionary and preparatory depression in the grief process of the terminally ill. In reactionary depression, immediate losses and changes are grieved. In preparatory depression, the ultimate loss of life is grieved. The chronically ill face both types of depression, but reactionary grief is the more frequent response, as flares and remissions require constant adaptation.

The big and small losses accumulated along the way in chronic illness result in a long-term grieving process. Your losses may include health, fantasies of immortality, privacy, control, role identity, independence, means of productivity or self-fulfillment, self-image, dreams or goals for the future, relationships, old ways of sexual expression, feeling good, undisturbed sleep, play or recreational activities, and energy, among many others.

The way you begin grieving your losses at the onset of your illness will influence how you go about grieving additional losses over the years. Research shows that people who actively grieve their diagnosis do better than those people who suppress, repress or deny the feelings of grief. Being able to moan, groan, cry and talk about the trauma of the diagnosis helped get the grief out of me and shrink my illness down to size, enabling me to go on with life.

Grief's Challenges

Grieving the losses associated with chronic illness has its own peculiar difficulties. You may be struggling with your own grief while also dealing with the mourning of your family. The first time Mother came to visit after my diagnosis, she embraced me and whispered, "Here's some of your grand-mother's jewelry. You might as well have it now," and "I'm glad the boys are as old as they are." I ran in stark terror.

However, the source of the grief process, you, is still present. You are a constant reminder to yourself and others around you of what's been lost.

After reacting to a diagnosis of chronic illness, your family faces a period of redefinition. In this process, the family's worldview is examined and reformulated. In much the same way that you need to synthesize and incorporate a new identi-ty, the family unit needs to also adopt one that accepts and understands your new circumstances.

During this family redefinition, some members' roles will change. You may have always been responsible, for example, for hosting big family get-togethers, where you cooked all your specialties, polished the silverware and made sure the entire house gleamed. Now others must help – or even replace – you. Or you may have always gone to every one of your chil-dren's ball games. Now it may be important for your husband or wife to take up that role. Men and women may find it dif-ficult to give up their primary roles.

In my own family, my roles as chief cook and bottlewasher at home, caretaker of my mother and source of a second income came to a crashing halt as I began to live my life from the bed to the couch to the hospital and back again. Major turmoil erupted.

My mother became weepy and clinging. My brothers seemed to get stuck in denial and it took quite some time to grasp that we would need to shift roles to take care of Mother, but eventually we did. My boys couldn't understand my limits and became frightened about my health, or overly occupied with their own health.

When it became clear I was seriously ill, everybody in my family pitched in – at first. Later, we hired a maid service to come in once a month to do the heavy house cleaning. The first day the maids came was like a funeral for me, even though I never relished doing housework. After I had to stop work, there was a long gap before we finally began to receive disability compensation. We came close to losing our house. Jim became depressed and angry.

The process of renegotiating and reformulating your new family image is a major transition. Your children or spouse may resent having extra responsibilities. You may resent losing them, along with the identity those responsibilities gave you as "provider" or "homemaker" or "problem-solver." But you may find that being "husband" or "mother" or "lover" does not necessarily depend on such abilities as bringing home a fat paycheck or making the perfect puff pastry.

Caution: Turbulence Ahead

The process of "becoming" can be turbulent. You may take two steps forward and three steps back. Through experience you and your family need to find new ways to replace your roles and functions within the family when you're in a flare.

Your family also needs to be flexible enough to allow you to reassume those roles during times of remission and feeling better. With time and love, your family, as a system, will come to understand how its meaningful relationships are affected by your altered capacity. Be patient: It is normal to take two to four years to grieve a significant loss that is stationary in time. My initial struggle took almost five years. The process will continue for the rest of my life.

You and your family may go through the grief process at different paces and in different ways. Allow each other to be different but together, separate but connected ... the true definition of intimacy.

Just as you experience problems accepting your diagnosis, your family will also go through denial, anger, bargaining and depression to get to acceptance. A problem arises when anyone in the family gets stuck at any one stage or phase of the letting-go process. You or they may cling to remnants of the old, highly valued memories of what your family used to be like and those unrealistic, mythical expectations of what your family should be.

Some families become trapped in a cyclic pattern of grieving and never make it through to acceptance and a new way of living. Those that do make it can find deeper, more meaningful relationships with healthier priorities for life.

Family members may not understand their or your continued mood swings and behaviors. You may become impatient with one another in your different stages of the process. The end result may be a build-up of tension between you and other members of the family.

This tension can plug into long-standing resentments, interfamily control issues, or anger from past wrongs. When there is no appropriate place to vent this anger, it may be directed within your family, causing more anger.

Unexpressed anger may cause some members of your family –

or you – to suddenly take immovable, differing points of view on almost anything and everything. How to spend limited resources of money and energy, discipline of children, chores around the house – all can become major battlegrounds.

Lack of communication about these issues prevents healing, weakens your family relationships, facilitates denial, and encourages behavior that avoids the problem. Counseling may help each family member become conscious of what the real issues are.

The Need to Grieve

Life is a highway, and you'll need to pay some tolls. If you try to run them, the consequences could be far more expensive than if you'd thrown your quarters in the basket when you came to it. In the same way, if you try to put off grief, you may well end up paying a higher price later than if you face it now.

If your illness occurs at a time when important tasks need to be taken care of, you may show little or no reactions at first. Grief may also be delayed if you feel the need to help maintain the morale of others.

Sooner or later, delayed grief will come out in your body or behavior. You may find yourself crying or depressed at every small goodbye to family or friends. You may be unable to sleep at night – or sleeping much longer than you ever had. You may lose friends. Sooner or later, you'll need to go through the pain and process.

It may take some time of living with chronic illness to actually determine the losses that are permanent and need to be grieved. When you do, the intellectual process may pave the way for the gut-level, heart-rending emotional process.

However, beware of thinking too long about your losses

without going through the pain. Over-intellectualization by itself may serve as a form of denial, allowing you to maintain a distance from messy and maybe frightening emotions. You need to progress to real grief before your emotional equilibrium can be restored.

As painful as they are, depression and tears will eventually help relieve your suffering. Grieving seems to lance the emotional wounds, allowing anger, bitterness, hurt and disappointment to be released. Without grieving, these emotional wounds may produce an emotional abscess – a more handicapping effect than the illness itself.

Physical changes from the illness, depression and the grief process can work together to perpetuate a cycle of grieving. Inactivity from a lack of motivation and loss of energy can lead to further physical losses (and even less motivation and energy). Health will be further diminished and depression deepened.

Letting go allows you to put the past in perspective, find meaning in the present, and develop coping strategies to go on with life. You will journey from an initial reaction of numbness and disbelief to a growing awareness of pain, sorrow, anger and preoccupation with what's lost. Gradually, you'll find reorientation, where the losses are accepted and balance is restored to your life.

You can't go forward looking back. Rebuilding and embracing life in the present is impossible until you let go of the past – but it's beautiful when you do.

Good Grief

Grief for your former life will act as midwife for the birth of the new you, as you are now. This grieving process may lend you valuable insights: You may find the essence of your own worth not overshadowed by the peripheral aspects of living and constant doing. Interests and talents you once had no time for may emerge, to be cultivated in the present.

You may develop new strengths as a byproduct of coping with chronic illness. You may treasure the gift of life more deeply, without conditions. You may become aware that you are a whole person, even in the midst of chronic illness.

Your grief may be reawakened when you suffer a relapse or flare, additional loss of ability, or failed treatment. Anniversaries of losses may be painful. But once you've learned how to process your grief, you'll handle each additional crisis better.

The Way We Weren't: "Fantasy Grief"

Not all grief is healthy. You may find yourself thinking of your former life and family as a romanticized version of "the way we were." Sometimes those mental pictures are really "the way we should have been": Perhaps during a lonely holiday you envision your whole, happy, healthy family gathered around the table at Thanksgiving, praying together before you serve the turkey.

The image may prove deeply painful if you're alone, or if you can no longer host such gatherings. But deep down, perhaps you also know that in fact such holidays were always crazy at your home, with your children sulking, your spouse absent and you yourself miserable because rigid, controlling Aunt Mildred has been there all day.

Still, those airbrushed family portraits may haunt your memory, and you'll find yourself grieving over that make-believe gathering or that "wonderful" time. Perhaps you reflect on what a great executive you were or how much you miss jogging, when really you hated your job and hardly ever exercised. Such feelings are called fantasy grief – not because the grief isn't real, but because the "memory" isn't.

People who come from a chaotic family of origin, or whose childhoods were very difficult, are more prone to fantasy grief, perhaps because they often fantasized to cope with difficult situations as they grew up. Recognize and label such feelings as fantasy. You'll have enough to grieve without them – and ill or well, it's never too late to create healthier more realistic relationships with your *real* family, or to be a person of worth as you are right now.

Finding Time for Grief

Mourn your losses on your own timetable. Grief can't be forced or pushed. Allow yourself plenty of time. As you embrace the totality of your experience, joy can evolve from the sorrow, laughter can push aside the tears, and peace can be found in the turmoil. The grief process can serve as a bridge between what used to be and what is now.

Grief will also help form scar tissue over the emotional wound your illness gave you. And as every nurse knows, scar tissue is stronger than normal tissue.

CHAPTER 3

Keys to the Process

The process of integrating your illness into your life can be long and difficult. The following ten key philosophies have helped me.

Key One: Accept and embrace the pain so you can exhaust it.

The urge to avoid grief's pain is natural. But how you deal with the process – whether you run from it or face it – is an expression of yourself. Quick solutions such as drugs, travel, hard work or a romance can be hollow. Blocking the pain and refusing to feel the grief can cause emotional wounds to fester.

The caterpillar's miraculous transformation to butterfly takes place inside its cocoon. The creature's entire structure is reorganized: Its parts break down and are put together in a different way to produce the butterfly. Its escape from the cocoon is an arduous struggle that forces fluids from its body into the butterfly's wings.

Without that struggle, the butterfly wouldn't emerge as a creature of delicate beauty, but with a bloated body and shriveled wings.

Similarly, in your integration process, the components of your life are broken down and organized in a different way. Your struggle to break out of your cocoon – and into another way of living – gives you the form of a new and different person.

Key Two: Experience the pain so you can release it.

Tears and courage are not opposites. As a matter of fact, they are closely related. To be yourself, allowing your feelings to come out, is to be courageous. Tears won't change your outward circumstances, but they will change you. Tears allow the release of emotions and may bring a new outlook to your life.

You can't release an emotion until you've fully experienced and processed it. Let the tears flow to cleanse your emotional wounds, thereby allowing healing and releasing you to move on in life. Unreleased emotions control you from the unknown of your unconscious and may cause more illness. This is a basic premise of trauma resolution therapy.

Key Three: Laugh. Try to see humor in your situation and *celebrate* life.

Grief and humor may be bound together because of the depth of the human problem and the desperate need to find some way of coping with it. Humor can shrink a problem down to a size so that you can then approach it. Laughter, fun and celebration are important aspects of life that can help you keep your illness in perspective.

The same muscle systems are used in both laughing and crying. Both bring relief from tension when done aerobically, using muscles deep down in your belly.

Key Four: Keep the lines of communication open with "I" statements.

Communicating clearly with others helps to bear the load, reflect reality, keep you on course and prevent defensiveness. Use "I" statements ("I'd like some help with the laundry") to avoid the accusation in "you" statements ("You never help with the laundry").

Facing and speaking your feelings, thoughts and needs allows you to connect with others and not feel alone. You share your burdens and multiply your joys.

Key Five: Seek out both moments of solitude and fellowship in your community.

Some people deal with their emotions by withdrawing from involvement with their world. When you separate yourself from your loving community, you may find you have sentenced yourself to loneliness.

Some panic at the thought of being alone and frantically seek out anyone and anything to fill their vacuum. But solitude can provide a center of quietness from which calm, wise judgments, opportunities for personal growth and creativity in living can emerge.

Key Six: Lean on your support people or get counseling to help find the way.

At times, you may be so close to your problems you won't be able to find your way through them. You may be able to see the pieces of the puzzle clearly, but may not know how to fit them together. Anger and depression in the integration process may get so heavy that you can't pull the load on your own. A set of fresh eyes – the perspective of a close friend or counselor – can help.

Key Seven: Take responsibility for yourself. You play a central role in your illness.

Those who seem to be the most angry tend to see themselves as victims and not as participants in their own lives. Assuming responsibility for yourself, mind, body and spirit is essential to moving beyond anger.

Key Eight: Reach beyond yourself by relying on faith.

Faith gives hope and courage to venture into the unknown. It is essential for stretching beyond your limits. Your belief in a higher power, whatever its expression, will inspire you to greater heights and achievements.

Key Nine: Live fully, even with a chronic illness.

Sometimes I've felt fully living with chronic illness presents a greater challenge than actually dying and leaving the daily battles and struggles behind.

Death is a breathing out of the spirit, perhaps requiring no effort or energy, but only a release. People living with chronic illness, more than others, need to come to terms with death or a shortened life span.

Acceptance in terminal illness means reaching a state of numbness and lack of feeling – a letting go of life. Acceptance of chronic illness includes dealing squarely with the little dyings and the threat of ultimate death. Rather than turning to the wall away from life, grieve your losses in order to wade back into life as a much different person.

The word "adjustment" is often used when referring to coping with a chronic illness, and "acceptance" used in reference to terminal illness. Both words can be summed up in the word "acknowledgment." Acknowledging your condition implies you have assessed your losses, found uniqueness in your experience and faced it squarely, and begun the search for new meaning in your life. At this point, you can integrate illness into your life as only a part of who you are.

Key Ten: Focus on expressing your uniqueness in your living, not in your dying.

Death and life go hand in hand. Everyone is going to die, regardless of the cause. The act of dying is the same release for everyone. Still, fear of death is one of the most basic and powerful human emotions, ingrained from early childhood.

All of nature is constantly in a flux of life and death. The cells in our bodies are continually dying and being replaced. In the fall, buds for new flowers and leaves are already on trees as leaves drop to the ground.

Even as your old self is dying, the potential for a new you grows within. What that new self will be is up to you. Reliable babysitter, financial expert, internet wizard, memoir writer, photo album organizer, jovial conversationalist or wily checkers strategist – your abilities and talents *as they are now* are unique and irreplaceable. Use them.

Take a moment now to think: What are some interests and passions you are free to explore now that your life may be slowing down?

The End-All and the Be-All

You can embrace life only after you have come to terms with your own small dyings, and ultimate death. Denying death gives you only a partial view of life. Fearfully and frantically clasping life only squeezes the *living* out of it.

On a roller-coaster ride, closing your eyes and desperately hanging on with a white-knuckle grip is painful. Throwing your hands in the air and screaming at the top of your lungs is thrilling.

A chronic illness may scare you to death – and cause you to give up living to the fullest. It may take a time of systematic desensitization to become comfortable with your illness. As the lyrics of the song "The Rose" go,

> *It's the heart afraid of breaking*
> *that never learns to dance.*
> *It's the dream afraid of waking*
> *that never takes a chance.*
> *It's the one who won't be taken*
> *who cannot seem to give.*
> *It's the soul afraid of dying*
> *that never learns to live.**

* From "The Rose" by Amanda McBroom. Copyright 1977, 1979 Warner Tamerlane Publishing Corp. All rights reserved. Used by permission.

As you have lived, so shall you die. What you become in the end depends on what you are trying to be right now. Eternity begins with the moment of now, is not permanence but significance, not duration but depth. Whatever your faith, may you find a new creative way of fully living that faces death squarely, then turns full face to live rejoicing in the celebration, of the gift of that life.

CHAPTER 4

Living with Chronic Illness

I was a visiting nurse, active in my career and moving up the promotional rungs, when I was knocked off my feet by health problems. Over a period of several years, I was diagnosed as having a chronic, up and down, incurable illness that could be fatal. The doctor's diagnosis coming over the phone that late Friday afternoon was like a deafening gunshot in my ears that echoed over and over.

Many years ago, a perfume commercial featured the "Enjoli woman," a sexy, smart and capable femme fatale who could do it all and still be desirable at the end of the day. Before the illness struck, that's how I often thought of myself, as I tried hard to be an ideal wife, mother, nurse, church member and community leader. As my old lifestyle of work, athleticism and involvement in the church faded, that image of myself slowly died. In fact, the Enjoli woman was knocked into such a deep hole I had a hard time crawling out. Instead, from my sickbed, I began thinking of myself as another, more anemic person: the Geritol woman.

For a long while, I was able to deny the long-term consequences of my condition, since my illness held the possibility of remission somewhere on the horizon. Disease activity would also fluctuate from time to time. During brief reprieves, my spirits would soar, only to be dashed as the pain, fatigue and nausea inevitably returned. Days stretched into weeks, weeks into months, and months into years.

My family and I kept taking the "old me" off the shelf, hoping one day she might return and we could go back to our past lives. We'd sigh and put her back on the shelf, but she lingered in our memories and hopes, thwarting any attempts of accepting and living in the present as it was. It was always, "Tomorrow we'll ..." or "Remember yesterday, when ...?"

One day I read an article in a rehabilitation magazine that compared the multitude of small deaths from chronic illness to ultimate death, and described the grieving inherent in each. At last I could identify the emotions I was experiencing: They were the stages of grief. The writer pointed out that the accumulation of these small deaths made ultimate death pale in comparison.

Ultimately, grieving my losses served as a bridge allowing me to celebrate my todays to the fullest, instead of being imprisoned in my yesterdays or tomorrows. Grief was the key that unlocked the door to my adjustment.

Barriers to Grief

Often society's response to the chronically ill is, "Just get over it! Get a grip! When will you straighten up and fly right?" You may try to accommodate these messages, but your illness is a fact you can't avoid.

Research results that I ran across in my master's program helped me understand that grieving is more difficult for the chronically ill than the terminally ill, because sporadic unpredictable remissions allow you to think you're really going to be all right. Perhaps it's also more difficult because there are no sanctioned ways of grieving small losses, unlike the familiar rituals of death. There are no wakes or black clothes to signal the significance of losing your health. Such barriers may postpone your eventual adjustment to a new life.

Assessing Your Losses

I slowly began to realize the enormity of what I had relinquished: my good health, nursing career, independence, sense of control, privacy, modesty, body image, relationships as they had been, self-image, family roles, social status, self-confidence, financial security, lifestyle, plans and dreams, fantasies of immortality, familiar daily routines, undisturbed sleep, sexual expression, leisure activities, getting a tan – the list could go on and on. I could only get on with my new life if I fully understood what was lost.

For me, the most difficult losses involved control over my life, sexuality and productivity. Those are thorny issues for many with chronic illness. Take a moment now and list things in the space provided that you feel you have lost due to your illness. Make it as long or as short as you want.

LOSSES LIST

Taking Control

After becoming ill, I lost the sense that I had control over my body and life. The realization shattered me. I was living in a body that had become a frightening stranger, and seemed to continually change, as I would feel okay one minute and lousy the next. I couldn't trust it anymore, or predict how it would respond to the demands I made on it.

I used to plan my life years in advance. Then it became difficult to make plans for even the next day. Daily I gave up new controls over my body and emotions, taking medication to help endure the effects of the disease. The medication would add its own strange effects, causing an even greater sense of helplessness and loss of control.

Fear of the illness itself, with its many unknowns, created a greater sense of loss of control. My sense of helplessness would bring on depression, adding to the depression that is sometimes part of the illness itself.

In his writings, psychiatrist and Nazi concentration camp survivor Victor Frankl compares the loss of control in a prison setting to that of a person imprisoned in his body by chronic illness. I found, as he did in his prison experience, that I could control my attitude, even if I couldn't control my circumstances.

I could let fear, anger or despair control me. On the other hand, I could take control of myself and choose to kiss the joy of each moment, tenderly caressing it and living it to the fullest, let it go, and then turn to the next.

Let's Talk About Sex

My grieving, as well as my illness, brought about changes in the way I expressed my sexuality. I learned that sexuality and sexual identity don't just involve sexual intercourse. You express your sexuality in the way you walk, what you wear, the way you do your hair, the roles you fulfill, and more.

Sometimes my illness identity and the grief process threatened to replace my sexual identity. I became "a lupus patient" rather than a woman who was sexy. The ways I expressed and reinforced my sexuality – like wearing high heels, dying and styling my long hair, wearing flimsy negligees, tanning myself in a sexy bikini – all needed to change.

In some ways, grieving the loss of the vanities connected with my hair loss, weight gain and sexuality were some of the most difficult. Putting on my cervical collar and clod-hopper orthopedic shoes did little to heighten my feeling of attractiveness.

Fatigue and pain aren't conducive to sexual arousal. And I

found the illness had brought about physical changes as well: Places on my body that had been erotic and produced sexual arousal in the past became tender, and off-limits. My old familiar ways of engaging in and responding to sexual arousal had changed.

Losing my work also affected my sexual appetite, since sexuality is an expression of the total being. The disability decree was also a blow to my self-confidence and self-esteem. You can only make love in a healthy way when you love yourself. I certainly didn't love myself with all these new strange changes.

My sleeping habits changed, and later a hospital bed invaded the bedroom. My husband and I were separated during hospitalizations. Family roles that defined sexuality roles needed to flip-flop as disease activity fluctuated between flares and feeling better. Jim assumed housekeeping and parenting roles, which he regarded as women's work, and then gave them back when I felt better. It all affected our sex life.

Communication is essential in a sexual relationship. It's important to head off erroneous assumptions about the illness that may lead you to drift apart. I found new ways of expressing and heightening my sexuality, sexual expression, sexual arousal and response that are more fulfilling than they have ever been.

Experimenting helped: Reading romantic novels or watching movies whetted my sexual appetite. I began developing a sexy new look that helped me feel better about myself. Our sex life improved when we cuddled and touched more. We experimented with new positions. I identified my own erogenous zones and what was pleasurable to me, sometimes using a vibrator or lubricants.

TALKING WITH YOUR PARTNER ABOUT SEX

Think about these questions and discuss them with your partner.

1. Has chronic illness altered your sexual relationship or your feelings about your sexuality?

2. What, if anything, has changed?

3. What is more or less the same?

4. Are there any sexual activities that are not as pleasant as they used to be?

5. Are there any that are more enjoyable?

6. Does lovemaking cause any special problems for you or your partner?

7. Where on your body do you enjoy being touched and what areas do you not wish to be touched?

8. Are there new things you would like to try? If so, what are they?

Adapted from "Sexuality and MS," National MS Society, 1983.

What You Are and What You Do

The loss of my career was one of the most agonizing areas of my life to grieve and let go. My work was an extension of who I was and what I valued about myself.

Perhaps even more difficult was the process of obtaining the official Social Security disability decree. I had always assumed that if you worked hard and did your best, things would work out. But now we were threatened with losing our home. Medical bills consumed us, and the threat of losing my insurance coverage loomed. After a year and a half of red tape, financial disaster and confusion, I took my place at the other end of the social structure. I had taken pride in myself as a productive citizen, and hated the long waits and humiliation of asking instead of giving.

This loss removed one of the most important means of control in my life. Gone were my income, productivity, self-expression, self-fulfillment, social outlet, identity and lifetime investment.

I did not know it at the time, but getting disability helped me create my new life as a writer, which I find as fulfilling as my work as a nurse. I could never come to love disability, but the payments stave off bankruptcy and I am thankful for the stability.

Take a moment now to list new talents and interests you've discovered since becoming ill.

DISCOVERY LIST

Losing Your Old Self

Of course, there is life outside of love and work. My avocations of singing, church involvement, outdoor activities and athletics were also difficult to give up. I'd pursued some of those interests since childhood.

I also forfeited activities that I had shared with my family, such as camping and vacations, that cemented us together. We needed to grieve these losses together as large portions of our old lives vanished and to find new ways to play together.

I sought value in my new state of being, devoid of the peripheral doings of life. In doing so, I discovered new ways of self-expression that reached out to others, incorporating my illness and disability identities as only a part of my total being, and discerning new ways to be part of my family and community.

New identities that have emerged are freelance writer, chaplain and counselor, among others. I can accept myself, warts and all. My illness is no longer all of my identity but integrated into my being as just a part of me. I couldn't embrace the "new me" until I had grieved, and put the "old me" on the shelf for good.

Grieving helped me get my present in perspective, not dwelling on the past or future. I could then develop coping strategies to make the most of the present. My emotional well-being no longer depended on my physical well-being. My body can be falling apart but my spirit can soar to heights I never knew possible.

Once the energetic Enjoli woman, and later the listless Geritol woman, I've now become the "Enjotol woman," who knows her limits but celebrates her abilities.

I have come to believe that in all the small deaths of chronic illness, ultimate death is the easy part. The breathing out of the spirit requires no effort. The real challenge lies in grieving my losses and then turning back to a life complicated by chronic illness, rejoicing in the daily celebration of the gift of that life.

CHAPTER 5

Denial

As discussed in Chapter 2, denial is often listed as the first stage of grief. However, many people with chronic illnesses may go through another stage first: relief. Some may have sought for years for the diagnosis they thought would bring answers, and briefly, but temporarily, find relief in hearing it. Often, however, that relief is fleeting. For many, the next stage is denial.

Denying your illness is a healthy unconscious defense mechanism when it keeps the impact of your illness from becoming overwhelming. It can allow you time to build your defenses while trying to figure out what you are up against and what to do next. It can also help prevent you from caving in to self-imposed limits that aren't necessary or realistic. In time, you need to move beyond denial. Getting stuck here can be dangerous.

Denial can take many forms: You may simply refuse to believe your diagnosis, however compelling the evidence. Your friends, family members and society may reinforce your denial, especially if the illness isn't physically visible. ("But you look so good!") Your own urge to be brave and strong and push through your illness, as well as society's mandate to do so, can also strengthen denial. If you're afraid of being left out of family or social activities, it may be difficult to not push yourself beyond what is healthy for you.

Experiments with laboratory animals find that behaviors reinforced irregularly and at unscheduled times are very tough behaviors to extinguish. Remissions in chronic illness can have the same effect because they reinforce denial irregularly and at unscheduled times. Feeling better for a few hours or days may throw you and your support people right back into denial, no matter how long you have lived with an illness.

Denial may go on for years or a lifetime. When in denial, you may be unable to observe individual patterns of your disease activity and learn how to respond to them. You don't listen to your body's signals. When in denial you may resist following your treatment plan.

I heard of one very ill lady who said, "I'm going to continue baking things the way I used to, even if it kills me." And it probably will kill her! Society applauds this kind of "heroic" approach. But such self-destructive behaviors seem pretty dumb to me.

Over-intellectualizing, another form of denial, can be a way of maintaining control. By over-intellectualizing your condition, you distance yourself from the pain of emotions, tears and depression. They are the very mechanisms that restore the grieved to normalcy. If you block the pain, your inner wounds will fester.

Denial, which Elisabeth Kübler-Ross links with isolation in *On Death and Dying*, may prevent you from asking for the help and support you need. You may become more and more detached from others and your own feelings.

When you cut off part of yourself with denial, you need to perform all the time to cover up the part of you that's missing. If you pretend with friends that you're not ill, you'll have to hide your symptoms when you're with them. This continual performance causes a great deal of stress that can stir up disease activity.

Denial can take the form of doing nothing – or taking up every activity possible. By throwing yourself into frenzied motion, you dodge the realities of your illness and put off grieving. Buying a new home, suddenly changing jobs, marrying or divorcing, shopping, traveling – all may be forms of denial that increase the family burden, and use up both financial and emotional resources needed to deal with the illness.

Denial is an unconscious, silky cocoon that protects you until you're ready to emerge. You can't move beyond denial until you're ready, and until you can cope with your condition. Don't try to strip away denial prematurely. It may be the only way to survive at the moment. Don't get stuck in denial. Once you've exhausted the need for denial, you'll be able to move from the no-man's-land between what was and what is to come.

Read through the list below and check where you think you may be with denial. Ask your significant others to do the same.

1. How do you use denial in a healthy way?
2. How do you use denial in an unhealthy way?
3. Do you perform to cover up your illness?
4. Do you simply think about your illness without experiencing your emotions?

CHAPTER 6

Anger

All emotions serve some purpose in your psychological make-up. It's what you do with them and how you express them that make them healthy or unhealthy. Anger is one of the most misused, misunderstood, but most valuable emotions in your repertoire. It's a signal you need to listen to, make sense of and act on.

You usually think of expressing anger in its extremes: wimpy avoidance or aggressive attack. Between these two is the assertive, kind, firm, clear, specific and direct expression of anger.

Chronic illness can provoke a great deal of anger in everyone it touches: patient, family and professionals. There is no suitable target for venting that anger, so health-care professionals often take the heat, since they are the closest at hand.

After all, they're the ones who pronounced the diagnosis, and they are a constant reminder of the illness that requires reliance and dependence on them. Anger may be directed toward the heavens, institutions, friends, family and self.

Anger can control you, causing physical decline and cutting you off from significant others. But handled in a healthy way, anger can be an important means of communication. Try to trace the real source of your anger. Anger can be connected more to childhood and issues from the past than what's happening in the present.

By understanding your anger, you can harness it and use its energy for change rather than letting it unconsciously control you. Proper channeling of this ever-present emotion can change your entire way of life, making it more comfortable and productive.

What Is Anger?

According to some popular theories, anger is a reaction to repressed childhood experiences, an expression of need, or an example of selfishness. None of these descriptions may be totally correct, but I see a common thread in each. Anger usually results when you feel unappreciated, belittled, taken for granted, helpless or in some way insignificant. Frustration or threats can also produce anger.

Triggered when an expectation is not met, anger can immobilize you. It is the result of wishing the world and people in it were different. When you are angry, you do not allow for variety, but demand that life and the people and events in it be a certain, prescribed way. You don't assume responsibility for yourself. Your external, physical world controls your internal, emotional world.

Anger that directly, clearly and specifically communicates personal needs with "I" statements, while also considering the needs of others, indicates a real strength. Selfishness can turn this constructive type of anger into a weapon. At times, you will need to argue your case, or even raise your voice to be heard. But if you bully others with a loud voice or consistent hostility, you will build a wall of resentment around youself.

You can't change anyone else. You can only change yourself. Your anger will only make others around you want to change you. The way you use your anger can make it a bridge for communication instead of a wall shutting others out.

Anger is a way of saying, "Notice my needs." You may displace feelings of anger and irritability on those closest to you. Family and friends may experience similar emotions and displace them on you. While trying not to express these feelings directly, they may unconsciously direct anger toward the patient. Or, in fact, they may be angry with themselves for being angry. Everyone may feel angry but be unable to address the real source: the illness.

Ideally, anger can actually help strengthen relationships. It's a sure sign that something needs to be changed. That can include your expectations of life, your unreasonable dependence on others, or the way you communicate with others. If you and those around you look at anger as an opportunity for constructive change, your adjustment to your new life will be smoother.

Sources of Anger in Chronic Illness

Chronic illness is certainly not something you wished for. Your life expectations may be shattered and replaced by something that you would never have dreamed of.

At the same time, expectations of your significant others may also have been blown apart, creating anger in all involved in your life. As chronic illness invades your life, your anger triggers may multiply.

Anxiety of a spouse or other family member involved in your care may cause anger and hostility to build between you. A struggle to show who's in charge or in control may develop.

A long-delayed diagnosis may also initiate anger – it's frustrating to seek answers and not find them. Once you get the diagnosis, anger may be stirred when medical health professionals can't offer assurances that everything will be all right or don't have all the answers. Mounting medical bills that accrue as illness continues can also irritate you, and dealing with a complicated health-care system can be downright maddening.

Anger is just one normal stage in the complicated passage of grief. When you get stuck in anger, you may unconsciously turn anger against yourself or others as part of your refusal to acknowledge the losses of self. In doing this, you give up living fully. Hopeless, you may become complacent in your anger or aggressively lash out at the world.

If you were already carrying anger from old hurts before you became ill, anger from the grief process may awaken it. Huge, angry blowups in response to small slights may have more to do with your past than your present.

Healthy people may aggravate you, especially when they complain about minor health problems, or abuse their health unnecessarily. They may only serve as another reminder of your severe losses. The chronically ill may have to remain silent, sharing their trials with only a special few.

Hopelessness, helplessness, fear and/or betrayal by the body add more fuel to the flames of anger. Limitations enforced by illness produce frustration and anger when they interfere with desired activities and necessitate dependency on others.

You may experience more frustration and anger when you are only marginally ill than when you are severely ill. It may feel as if you have one foot in the world of the sick and the other in the world of the healthy.

There may also be resentment and anger on the part of the person who has your needs thrust on him. Initially, anger may be caused by interference from well-meaning helpers. Their efforts to help may seem demeaning and be interpreted as pity or a lack of confidence in your ability to handle things on your own.

Later on, when you are tired and need help, it may not be offered. Anger may brew because others may not be sensitive enough to recognize your need for help or read your mind. You'd rather it be given without having to ask, since this may feel demeaning.

Anger can be born from all these unique things that go with chronic illness, adding to the accumulation of the normal, everyday frustrations. When you're already angry, you tend to have a short fuse. Feeling ill doesn't make you the most cheerful person in the world. If you are chronically ill, expect to be angry from time to time.

What's at Stake

Anger is a common response to separation and loss. Physical illness or disability can often bring on dysfunctional anger, at least initially. This is because, at first, there is a sense of disbelief that the losses of the self and others are permanent. As permanence becomes a reality, anger is an effort to signal the return of what's lost.

But in fact, angry, aggressive behavior tends to alienate and drive significant others away, rather than bring them closer or bring your health back. When suffering loss frequently, your anger may seem selfish and irrational. Yet it's understandable.

In the early phase of chronic illness you frequently question your worth. You may want people around you to reassure that they still like and need you even if you are ill. Anger works against maintaining old essential relationships and forging new ones.

Within relationships, an anger/guilt/depression cycle may evolve. You may feel guilty and depressed because of your anger and become angry over your guilt and depression.

Even if you attempt to hide, repress or deny your feelings, they are likely to be expressed in some way. You may display your anger through manipulation or excessive demands. Fear of expressing your anger may cause you to be compliant or agreeable. Your anger will find a way to come out in your body or behavior if you don't talk about it and process it. Pent up anger associated with unwisely managed grief may show up in how you relate to others, unhealthy emotional patterns, and physical manifestations.

You may turn your anger outward, blaming others for your illness or your failure to improve. On the other hand, you may turn your anger inward, blaming yourself for your condition and feeling guilty for causing yourself and others so much trouble and expense.

Your anger may be linked with an effort to find something, someone or anything to blame for your illness – the eternal "why." You may try to explain your illness by irrationally linking mysterious events.

At the same time, old familiar physical outlets to get your anger out of your body may be decreased because of physical limitations. The loss of your former outlets may create even more anger as you lose yet another pleasure in your life.

Suicide may be a real threat during periods of anger as well as depression. Seek professional help immediately if you are experiencing thoughts of harming yourself or anyone else.

As you acknowledge and live with your illness, the anger – yours and loved ones' – will become less pervasive. You may experience a period of reconciliation and reconstruction, as new realities are tested out and relationships mended. As you become more at peace with yourself, you will be more at peace with those around you.

Handling Anger

There is no one correct way to handle anger. You can repress it, suppress it, express it or release it. Each style contains its own pitfalls and dangers.

Repression

Repression is an unconscious defense mechanism in which an unwanted feeling is pushed into subconscious. You can consciously stuff feelings that threaten you. You may try to repress your anger out of fear of alienating others, or as a form of denial. If you deny that you're angry, you don't need to deal with it, but it doesn't go away.

Repressed anger can be dangerous, since it can fester in the subconscious, becoming powerful and bitter. Once anger is pushed into the subconscious, it is out of your immediate control. Excessive irritability, quarreling, and even tense and sore muscles may result.

Suppression

Suppression is a conscious attempt to hold back or block anger. Holding anger in without expressing it healthily may lead to a blowup. However, at times, suppressing anger is a healthy choice. When you're in pain, you may find yourself easily irritated. Unhappy with being cooped up in the house, you may snap at others. In such cases, a little suppression to process that anger at a later time is healthy. Such old-fashioned exercises as counting to 10, or taking a deep breath, or simply holding your tongue from an immediate retort can save a lot of wear and tear on relationships.

Expression

Anger can be expressed in many ways, verbally and nonverbally. Much anger may be expressed in passive-aggressive ways that tend to cut off any means of healthy, open communication. Anger may be seen in passive resistance to treatment and measures to improve your health. Somehow, you just can't follow that medication, diet, rest or exercise regimen.

Doctor-shopping may be a sign of repressed anger that has resulted from not finding a doctor who agrees with you. Sarcasm, chronic complaining and stubbornness all may be means of holding onto anger, giving you a sense of power over others.

Silence can be a potent expression of passive-aggressive anger, and is perhaps the most effective weapon you can use to control others. Procrastination, another form of passive-aggressive anger, may also be an attempt to control. Constant depression may be a passive means of saying that you feel the world is no good, a cover for anger, or the result of anger.

A well-ingrained pattern of forgetfulness, preoccupation, laziness, hypochondria, verbal outbursts, gossiping, intimidation of others and ruminating incessantly can be subtle expressions of anger that prevent the honest communication of feelings.

GOOD AND MAD: HEALTHY EXPRESSION

In everyday communication, rules to guide the constructive expression of anger include:

1: Don't try to establish your superiority or claim special privileges because of your illness.
2: Consciously, choose a constructive aim or goal for expressing your anger rather than unconsciously reacting and blowing up aggressively.
3: Be sensitive to the person you wish to communicate with, and notice his or her responsiveness. Some people may never be responsive to you or your situation. Choose your battles wisely.

At times, some things may be better left unsaid – when, for example, the person you're talking to is already depressed. Picking times when a person seems the most open to you can make all the difference in the world.

Since those who are intimately interwoven with your care may also be experiencing anger, establishing communication channels outside your immediate circle of family and friends may be helpful and even vital in blowing off excess steam and emotional energy.

You can probably express your anger more honestly to someone who is not so caught up in your immediate situation. But also let that person know that you are aware of heaping your problems on him so he will know you are sensitive to his needs.

Release

Chronic illness may hamper ways to release anger. Jogging, walking, swimming or any physical activity may not be feasible anymore. Losing these outlets for tension may evoke even greater anger. Find new ways to work off your tension. Try opening your window and yelling at the top of your lungs. Stereophonic, creative, aerobic crying while beating a pillow helps. Sing loudly. Exercise – if you stay within your limitations or level of fitness – is a great way of working off steam and strengthening your body at the same time. What helps one person may not help another. The activity needs to be aggressive in nature but not directed at the person you're angry with.

Relationships suffer, and peace and laughter will be blocked until you experience, express or release your anger. You remain a constant slave to your anger when you refuse to accept responsibility for deciding your own destiny. You can be both "good" and "angry" at the same time. The way you handle anger ultimately reflects your level of health and how you feel about yourself.

Once you release anger, you no longer need it. You can release anger only after you have learned how to recognize it, experience it, process it, express it and use it constructively to build relationships.

Check your level of anger with these questions:

1. What are sources of anger for you? List them.
2. What are ways that you used to vent anger that you can no longer do?
3. What other emotions might you be feeling that come out as anger (such as fear, hurt or guilt)?
4. Who are the innocent bystanders that you turn your anger toward who don't really deserve to be blasted?
5. How do you process, express and release your anger? Are your methods healthy? List and rate them as healthy or unhealthy.

CHAPTER 7

Bargaining

Like any stage of grief, bargaining can also be a healthy passage unless you get stuck in it. Bargaining is the stage of the "ifs": "If I do this or that, I'll be okay." "If I'm 'good,' I won't be sick." Of course, your illness doesn't work that way.

Bargaining is also the stage of shopping for every medical treatment, diagnostic test and doctor's opinion available. You may subconsciously seek a diagnosis or explanation that you like better. It's really a search to reclaim the lost parts of life. Certain species of geese who mate for life go through a similar search when their mate dies. For a year, they return to every place they have been with their mates to look for them.

It's important to strike a balance between giving up the search and making it your whole life. Always be on the lookout for ways to take care of yourself and be healthy, but don't let it consume you.

I have watched people flit from one "magic answer" to

another. When one method doesn't work, they abandon it in search of the next instant cure. It probably took many things together for you to get sick. It'll take many things together to get you better. Look for a holistic approach that includes many strategies. Introduce one new strategy at a time and give it weeks or months to see if it helps, and keep what works for you.

Constantly continuing the search may keep you from settling in with one doctor and hammering out the best treatment for you over time. You may exhaust your financial, physical, and emotional resources. Or you may reach your optimum level of health, but keep searching so that you can't fully live in the "now."

Check the list below to see where you may be with bargaining.

1. Are you constantly searching to find that magic cure for your condition?
2. Have you given up on improving your health in other ways?
3. How much do you spend on unproven remedies that might keep you from other needed medical care?
4. Do you live in the present, or are you focused on the future, when you may find that dream of a cure?
5. Do you feel angry when you've rested, taken your medicine and done all the things you're supposed to do and still don't feel like your old self?

CHAPTER 8

Depression

The World Health Organization lists clinical depression as the world's most widespread disease. Studies show that people with chronic illness experience depression that is more severe and more frequent than the rest of the population.

Reactive depression is in response to an event or circumstances in your life. It is a part of the grief process and sadness about loss. Clinical depression is a serious medical illness that affects the mind and body. Psychological, biological and genetic factors contribute to its development.

Clinical depression isn't a condition that you can just pull or will yourself out of. You need medication and counseling.

The signs and symptoms for both kinds of depression are similar. The difference is in the intensity and duration of the symptoms and how severely they affect your ability to function. For the most part, I'll be talking about reactive depression in this chapter. Some portions can apply to clinical depression, too.

SIGNS/SYMPTOMS OF DEPRESSION

- A persistent sad, "empty" or anxious mood
- Loss of interest in ordinary activities (such as grooming, hobbies, work, sex); isolation/withdrawal from people
- Decreased energy, fatigue, feeling "slowed down"
- Trouble sleeping or changes in sleep patterns
- Increased or decreased appetite/weight gain
- Difficulty concentrating, remembering, making decisions; frequent accidents
- Feeling hopeless, pessimistic, unusually discouraged
- Feeling helpless, like a failure, guilty, worthless; low self-esteem/self-image
- Frequent arguments or loss of temper; restlessness
- Excessive crying
- Thoughts of death or suicide; suicide attempts

Your chronic illness and the medications you take can cause several of these symptoms. However, you should seek professional help if you have symptoms that last for more than two weeks and are severe enough to disrupt your daily life. If you have suicidal thoughts, seek professional help immediately!

Reactive depression is shifting emotional energy. Don't medicate or avoid this kind of depression. Ride it like a horse. It will take you somewhere and teach you something about yourself. You don't get over depression but get through it. It can be the road out of the grief process.

Depression isn't a sign that you've somehow failed. It is, instead, a message and signal from your body and psyche. It may be a sign that your expectations of yourself or others are unrealistic.

You may push your emotions to the back of your mind so you can cope with a crisis. After the immediate crisis passes, those emotions may come rushing to the fore. Thus it is usually when you are able to relax and look back that you are most likely to be hit the hardest by depression.

If depression is your constant frame of mind, you may require counseling or medication. Depression can feed on itself, producing more depression, if it is not recognized, labeled and dealt with.

My one brief encounter with clinical depression was a real eye-opener. It's much more severe and incapacitating than reactive depression. Whether your depression is mild or severe, the first step is actively recognizing it and saying to yourself or to someone else, "I am depressed." I'd rather go through anything physical than experience clinical depression again.

Depression can make pain and fatigue worse. Fatigue can intensify pain and depression. Pain can magnify depression and fatigue so that you get into an endless cycle. Pain, fatigue and depression can interfere with sleep cycles, once again complicating the whole picture.

Once depression is acknowledged and labeled, you can do something about it. Keep in mind that you alone are ultimately responsible for taking care of yourself. No one else can do it for you. Others only serve as encouragement or as guides. Reactive depression or sadness is a part of a normal cycle that all human beings go through, and is to be expected when you're chronically ill. Don't let it throw you.

However, if you find yourself thinking of harming yourself or others, get help immediately. Someone with a chronic illness is more likely to carry through on thoughts of suicide than someone with a terminal illness. The demands of constant struggle with the pain, fatigue and depression of ongoing illness may deplete your resources to keep facing life.

Keys for Dealing with Depression

Key One: Allow yourself to experience and exhaust the pain of loss. Don't fight it or belittle yourself for being sad or depressed. Know it's part of a process and need not last forever.

Sadness isn't all bad. Sometimes it's a kind of luxury. You may need a break from being cheerful, brave and having everything under control. It may give you a chance to catch your breath. You may have spent a lot of energy denying your anger and guilt.

In the cycle of adjustment, you may experience anger, denial, bargaining, depression and acceptance. Sadness may be hitting the wall of reality, experiencing the pain and tears, letting it all hang out. If you never experience depression, you may be stuck in another stage of integrating the illness into your life.

Key Two: Examine your feelings to determine what might be causing your feelings of loss or sadness and depression.

Sadness can cover other potent emotions that you may not want to own up to, like anxiety, anger and guilt. Recognizing depression as a cover for other emotions may help you look beyond it to see what's there.

Key Three: Get to know yourself, your thoughts and what triggers your depression.

When you're depressed, your thoughts can wander aimlessly. Writing things down can help you think more logically and lead you out of confusion. Once when I was really depressed, I sat down and listed everything I was angry about.

I found out there were about two dozen things. I was even angry about being angry. List the things you may feel angry, guilty or anxious about. You may begin to understand your thoughts and feelings better.

Depression in chronic illness may come from many sources – the illness itself, reaction to the illness and its effects, side effects from drugs, or reaction to life events or people. When depression hits, try to determine if you're reacting to an event. But also take a look at your medications, pain and fatigue levels to see what may be feeding what.

Key Four: Go ahead and have a good cry.

Don't be ashamed to cry creative, stereophonic, aerobic tears. Cry yourself a river, a lake or an ocean. Tears can be a cleansing, healing bath that washes away hurt and pain. Catharsis and complete release of an emotion are common ingredients in the healing practices of native cultures.

Strangely enough, one salty teardrop rolling off a cheek can carry the weight of many emotions. Research has shown that emotional tears take part in an eliminative process in which they actually remove toxic substances and chemicals that build up during stress. They may be important in the maintenance of physical health and emotional balance. Crying is a way of getting through your grief. Chemical analysis of tears shows they contain substances that build up during stress. Crying can help to remove those stress chemicals from the body.

If you find you can't cry, you may need to deliberately seek something out that will get the tears rolling. Rent a good tear-jerker, or listen to that beautiful, sad ballad. Reading or writing can also get the tears going.

Sometimes, crying by yourself is what you need. Crying with someone else can also be cleansing. The family that cries together may stay together. I am more concerned about someone who doesn't cry than someone who does cry. How much you need to cry depends on you, but certainly if you cry nonstop for weeks, you may be clinically depressed and need to consider getting help with your depression.

If over the period of a few months, you don't find yourself swinging back and forth between tears and periods of relief, you may need counseling to make sense of what the tears are all about.

Key Five: Regular exercise, within your level of fitness, may help break the chronic depression/fatigue cycle.

Research shows that exercise can help relieve depression. Circulation is stimulated to carry off wastes, and oxygen is carried to brain cells.

If you've ever awoken feeling exhausted after a full night's sleep, you've experienced the hallmark symptom of depression. Sleep cycles may be disturbed with depression, creating more fatigue and depression. Exercise can tire the body, often producing better sleep. See Chapter 25 for more benefits of exercise.

Key Six: Your depression may worsen during winter months, when you're confined inside, or on rainy days. Open your curtains and raise your shades to let the light in!

Research also shows that the cycles of night and day are reflected in bodily and emotional cycles. Depression seems to be more prevalent in the winter months, when there is less light. Patients with pathological depression have shown improvement when exposed to longer cycles of bright light.

Key Seven: Good nutrition and a balanced diet may slow or even reverse a downward spiral of depression.

"You are what you eat": If you're not feeling up to cooking, you may rely on junk food. But chips and candy will only make you feel worse. Learn simple, nutritious, well-rounded recipes or buy prepackaged but healthful foods, and limit snacks to fresh fruits and vegetables and foods high in carbohydrates.

Key Eight: Identify your key support people and let them know when you need them.

Seek out special people who can be a support and whom you can ask for help. It's often one of the most difficult things to do – admitting you can no longer make it on your own. Share your situation with those people. They may not end up being the people who are closest to you. Just remember that you need more than one person with whom to share your load to provide a broad base of support.

Key Nine: Plan an activity or treat that you really enjoy for those days when you are most prone to depression.

Certain dates or times of the year may be more difficult than others. Birthdays, anniversaries of good and bad times and holidays are potent with emotions. Mark those times in red on your calendar, and plan something fun and nourishing to occupy your mind. Be aware of your limitations and plan accordingly: Have some people over, see three movies in a row or go with a friend to a concert or that new restaurant you've heard about or order in if you can't get out.

Key Ten: Establish schedules, write down things you need to do, and check them off when done. Stay involved with others, whether by mail, phone, e-mail, newspapers or television.

With the onset of illness, a very active life may come to a standstill. You may have lost the structure of your life provided by a schedule. Idleness may replace activity, boredom may drown vitality, and an all-consuming preoccupation with the self may push aside interest in life.

These occurrences may create a fertile climate for depression. If part of getting sick is focusing on the self, then part of getting well is focusing outside the self.

Key Eleven: When experiencing increased pain and/or depression, try to differentiate between them. They sometimes go hand in hand. Treat the problem from both directions, as pain and/or depression, and see which approach works best. Both entities can make the other worse.

When you're depressed, you often focus on the internal functioning of your body. Any symptom, ache or pain may become magnified and intensified beyond its realistic significance. Pain and other bodily complaints can mask depression, since all attention may be focused on the physical problem.

Rather than wallowing in or getting stuck in depression, you can experience and exhaust it, educate yourself about it, and use it as a constructive phase. Growth, insight, breaking down walls, opening doors and developing sensitivity for life and those around you can occur. It's what you do with it that makes it healthy or unhealthy.

Like any other cycle of grief, depression is useful and healthy, if it's just another part of your journey. But if it becomes a long-standing haven, reach outside yourself for help.

See where you are with depression.

1. Do you cry too much, not enough, or not at all?
2. Are you afraid that if you cry and give in to the pain that you'll be washed away?
3. What medications are you taking that might add to your depression?
4. Do you get caught in any of these depressive cycles:
   • anger, guilt, depression, anger
   • disease activity, fatigue, pain, anger, depression
   • depression, guilt
   • pain, lack of sleep, medication, depression
5. Do you ever think of suicide, tried to commit suicide, or have a plan of how you might try to commit suicide?

CHAPTER 9

Acceptance

Some people think of acceptance or integration of a chronic illness as either complete capitulation or total vigilance. Actually it is neither. Acceptance is, in reality, an integral part of life. You accept a gift, a compliment, a job offer, someone's love, a challenge.

To accept is defined as "to receive or take in, hold or contain." Another definition refers to acceptance as "being done willingly or gladly." Acceptance of a chronic illness, however, is done out of necessity. Capitulation for the chronically ill means surrendering identity to the illness. Healthy acceptance incorporates an element of defiance, as you refuse to become a useless person even in the face of declining health. Acceptance allows you to become more than your illness. Do what you need to take care of you, and reinvent yourself.

Some signs of acceptance include:

1. You no longer focus on your illness or yourself. For a while this focus is necessary, but eventually, as you reach acceptance, the illness becomes only a part of your life and not its overriding concern. Sometimes your illness can become your god or the main focus of your life rather than just a guide.

2. You begin to see the needs of and reach out to others again. You may feel you are unique and that no one's problems can equal yours, but as you acclimate to your illness, your preoccupation with yourself will subside and you will feel empathy for others' situations.

3. The illness is only a part of your total identity. You no longer consider yourself just a (whatever) patient, so you don't feel compelled to tell everyone about your latest medical milestone.

4. You don't need to hide your illness. Acceptance requires that you absorb it within your psychological outlook in such a way that it is no longer a painful fact that must be concealed. Trying to hide or forget something is the best way to remember it, and it uses up a lot of emotional and physical energy.

5. You learn to handle the illness' effects so they do not contaminate every part of your life.

6. You identify with people who have similar conditions.

7. Your life is well-rounded, with many interests from your old life and the new.

8. You've accepted your condition intellectually and emotionally. Over-intellectualization may be a form of denial. But intellectual acceptance may lead the way to emotional acceptance.

9. You no longer think of yourself as a victim but as a participant in your illness who is in control and responsible for yourself. Feelings of bitterness, defensiveness and anger are released.

10. Your fears turn from generalized, consuming anxiety to more realistic concerns.

11. You acknowledge your limitations and learn to ask for help in an assertive way. Aggression, whimpering or complaining are not helpful tools for bargaining with your limitations.

12. You see humor in your situation and learn to laugh and play again.

13. You set new goals when old ones are no longer realistic.

14. You feel hopeful again. Those hopes are no longer unrealistic scenarios, but possible, reachable achievements – if you stretch for them.

15. You see yourself as being no different from others, only as an average Joe. You find similarities with the struggles of others, whether they're sick or well. You've decided to cast off the sackcloth and ashes – you're not a martyr or saint, just someone who's handling your problems as well as possible.

16. You see yourself as a person of value as you are right now. Acceptance is an everyday see-saw and balance. Part of you wants to get on with life as it is now and another part wants to stay with the loss. Accepting a chronic phasic illness can be like trying to hit a moving target while riding a roller coaster.

Balancing it all out takes a lot of time, patience, love, determination and understanding. Only through acceptance of your life as it is now can you discover peace and joy.

Acceptance implies a refusal to let your illness control you. You accept yourself as you were, let go and then turn to reinvent yourself – integrating all of who you are now.

PART II

Relating to Yourself and Others

CHAPTER 10

The Secret of Living in the Present

As people journey through life, they come across secrets that ease their burdens. Those who carry extra burdens, such as chronic illness, may be even more attuned to finding these secrets.

I've come across two secrets in my journey with chronic illness: present-moment living and realistic hope. I discover more about these concepts every day. I've even learned that present-moment living, which I initially wrote about from hard-earned experience with illness, has been used for years in 12-step recovery programs (such as Alcoholics Anonymous and Overeaters Anonymous).

Present-moment living and realistic hope may seem somewhat contradictory, but really, each concept supports the other. And they are both essential.

One Day at a Time

When I became ill, I felt I'd dropped off the end of the earth into an entirely new, fog-engulfed existence. I was consumed with fear of the future, and longed for my familiar, comfortable old life.

Slowly, paths to my new life began to emerge, but I found myself rendered immobile, imprisoned by the bars of yesterday and tomorrow. Simply trying to survive, I prayed to make it through a single day. I focused on one moment at a time.

I forced myself not to dwell on the past and future, but to concentrate on my todays. I found that taking one moment, one hour, one day, one step, one task at a time freed me to experience and enjoy where I was in the "now".

Often, I would slip back into my old patterns and would need to will myself back to the day-by-day, moment-by-moment frame of mind. I realized that I couldn't control what thoughts came into my head, but I could control what I did with them. I could either focus and obsess on them, deliberately block them out and concentrate on something else, or process and release them.

All we really have any certainty about is the present moment. You can combat immobilization by learning to live in it. Getting in touch with your "now" is at the heart of effective living.

That precious, present moment is tarnished and wasted if you constantly invest your energies and hopes in the future: toward that goal, that remission or that magical time when things might get better. Some choose to dwell in a future that looms ahead as a great, feared unknown.

Clinging to the glories, the hurts, the resentments or the guilt from the past can also be confining. Live as you are, where you are, not where you used to be in the past or as you hope to be in the future.

Victor Frankl, a psychiatrist who survived a Nazi concentration camp, observed that you can't always choose your circumstances, but you can choose your attitude toward those circumstances.

For me, present-moment living slowly evolved from a survival tactic to a means of celebrating the abundant life ... embracing "the goods" and "the bads." It is the ultimate in living and experiencing all of life, whether you are confined to bed or not.

There is something of beauty and value in every moment, no matter what our situation. A relationship, an inner sense of peace and joy, the unending beauty and drama of nature, the sheer determination to stick things out, a total awareness of all about us, deciphering a doubt, discovering a truth – all are worthy of celebration.

Little by little, month by month and year by year, fear and mourning loosened their chokehold on me so I could venture out into life and risk once again.

Gradually, cautiously, I allowed myself to emerge from the safe cocoon I had wrapped myself in to wade back into life as a totally different person. I had needed that protection to ready myself for this new life. Like a butterfly, I ventured forth as a much-changed creature – fragile, but stronger than I appeared, and beautiful in a much different way. I was now far more aware of myself, of life and of others. I knew what it was to die and be reborn.

I am still trying to learn how to totally experience and gently kiss the joy of my present moments, as if they were lightly floating butterflies, and to lovingly let them take their places in the past as others replace them. To cling too tightly to them would crush and destroy them.

The elusive present moment that comes and goes in a flash can be most beautifully experienced if you let yourself get lost in it. Drink in each moment with every sense. Tune out the past that is over and done with and the future that'll arrive in its own good time. Embrace this very moment with everything in it (joy or sorrow, laughter or tears, pain or ease) as the only time you really have.

Millisecond Victories

In going through the uproar of divorce, school, illness and launching teenage sons, I found that making it one millisecond at a time was a glorious victory! I was bedbound during the 1996 Olympics after one pretty radical surgery. Flat on my back, I watched the Games on television. Event after event was repeated in super-slow motion, showing how one athlete's victory and another's defeat was measured by the millisecond.

I too was moving in slow motion – or barely moving at all. My Olympic event for the day might be making it to the bathroom or just sitting up. The glory of victory ... the agony of defeat ... millisecond living! I certainly wouldn't have passed a drug test for steroids!

Many days I found myself with great effort fumbling, stumbling, falling and crawling through the day on my knees – living by Braille. Focusing on one task at a time gave me sanity. If I looked at the whole mess, I was done in even before I started. I tried to break each day down into reasonable manageable tasks and celebrate each victory in the moment.

A quote from Robert Raines' book *To Kiss the Joy* (1977)

became my motto for living. "To kiss the joy of life (a delicate butterfly) as it flies is to live in the Spirit. It is to live boldly immediately with gracious abandon daring to risk much, willing to give oneself. It is to live in unison with our dream; to see the sun shining in the smallest creatures; to create the marvelous by contagion" (p85).

See where you are with living in the present.

1. Describe where you are in your life at this very moment. (Examples: "I am a legal secretary with diabetes." "I am moving and am very stressed-out about it." "I've just lost my job." "I'm struggling for identity." "I am a mother who is no longer able to care for my kids." "I am always sad and can't seem to reach out to my family.")
2. What is the next step or task after this moment? (Examples: Brushing your teeth, combing your hair, getting dressed, eating breakfast, crying.)
3. What has been a millisecond victory for you recently? (Examples: Sitting up, getting up, sleeping through the night, running an errand.)
4. How did you celebrate it? (Examples: Called someone to share a victory, ate a Snickers bar, gave a whoop of joy.)

CHAPTER 11

The Secret of Hope

One of the first signs of adjusting to a crisis is the awakening of hope. Though you may still feel depressed at times, once you begin to feel hopeful, you may begin to reconstruct your life; gain appreciations and concepts; set new goals; and be able to minister to others.

The present is beautiful and stretches beyond the limits of the past and the future. Once I'd discovered the secret of living in the present, that became my hope. But then I realized that hope for present-moment living wasn't enough. I needed goals that reached out into the future, too.

Hope can't be reasoned or bought. Nor can it be swayed by logic or thought. Hope cannot be summoned up at will, but can survive the most difficult circumstances. Hope is just a small spark of light, but its beacon illuminates the future, and gives life meaning and direction.

Hope guarantees nothing, but provides strength and

endurance. Hope is powerful – it can actually change the physiologic state of your body. A chain reaction occurs, with hope as a catalyst, that results in a healthier balance.

Hope may play a part in the placebo effect, a well-known phenomenon in medicine. In experiments, patients were given pills for their aches and pains. Many reported relief, even though the pills were made of sugar.

Hopelessness also has an effect on the body. The immune system is weakened during severe depression, limiting its ability to handle infections and cancer. Loneliness produces similar results.

When coupled with positive expectations, hope can help relieve pain and improve your mental and physical health.

Real Hope

Your hopes need to fit within the confines of reality if they are to help rather than harm you. Victor Frankl, the psychiatrist and concentration camp survivor, observed that fellow prisoners who set unrealistic deadlines for release withered and died when those dates came and passed without freedom.

Professionals in rehabilitation medicine aim for patients' goals to be attainable, and increasingly difficult. If unrealistic goals are set and the patient fails, hope is dashed and progress is hampered. Meeting one goal breeds hope for more difficult ones.

Realistic hope accepts what is, without eliminating the possibility of what might be. Recognize your limitations and explore your strengths.

My hope began with accepting myself as a valuable human being whether I was in the hospital or lying on the couch. Because of my limitations, I could no longer maintain my old means of employment, but I could be home when my boys came in from school. I could learn from reading or enjoy listening to music. I could experience and enjoy everything in the present moment.

I didn't know until I fell ill that I could write or that I had a talent for listening to and encouraging others. I've seen other people in my support groups find talents as artists, a passion for singing, or new ways of expressing who they are that benefit others.

As you adjust your expectations to fit your new circumstances, your hopes may change. Your goal of doing great things may change to just being faithful in the moment to what's at hand. You may find yourself becoming a "human being" instead of a "human doing." My hope before I got sick was to be successful at everything I did. My sense of "being" came from that doing.

Since I became enrolled in the school of living with illness on a daily basis, I have found that I need to let my "doing" be an overflow of my "being," not the reverse. My involvements need to spring from a passion within me. I've learned to live from the inside out, not the outside in. I am not what I do. My "doing" is only an extension and a reflection of who I am. Operating this way puts me at ease with myself.

When I reached the stage in my master's-level counseling program where I was to do my practicum and internship, it looked totally hopeless that I could physically carry it off. I was devastated. Finally, I realized that the master's degree didn't define who I was, but would only be a reflection of who I was already!

As an expression of that understanding, I had 1,000 business cards made up declaring I was a "Specialist in Living with Chronic and Terminal Illness." (And later, I earned the degree.)

I have followed one breadcrumb of hope at a time to take me where I am at this moment.

Following Hope

As I emerged from crisis to acceptance, I remember feeling hopeful for the first time. It felt as though hope sprang up like a tulip in springtime from the dark hard earth to the promise of warmth and light. New thoughts began to bud, new dreams were born, and new directions presented themselves in the perfect timing of the seasons of my life.

It was tempting to ignore, run away from or thwart these fragile, budding promises of life. With them was an attendant threat of further disillusionment, lost dreams, failure and pain. I could argue away these tentatively hopeful thoughts, or listen to their whisperings of things to come and haltingly follow their call one step at a time.

I find myself swinging back and forth between despair that my life will never be any better and hope for a brighter tomorrow. My spiritual connection and faith alone give me the strength to walk into the unknown void of my future.

At times I stumble, stagger and lose my way, but determinedly, patiently and tenaciously, I whistle in the dark and make slow, forward motion. One step and task leads to the next, and I am overjoyed and awed as I look back and see that my footprints have been leading somewhere and not just aimlessly wandering.

CHAPTER 12

The Big Question

How are you?" It was once a simple question, one you've probably asked and answered without thinking thousands of times. But after you become chronically ill, these few words can begin to represent a huge dilemma. You can answer only after carefully weighing many factors. When the reply is no longer an automatic "Fine," the result can be a delicate moment for both the questioner and the questioned.

Learning how to answer that common, but critical, question is a big step toward learning how to relate to others after you've been diagnosed with a chronic illness. I'm convinced that dealing with a spouse, children, family, friends, professionals and casual acquaintances is one of the hardest parts of being sick! Understanding the complex forces behind this everyday exchange, as you and those around you adapt to your condition, will help. The key is becoming comfortable with yourself just as you are. After that, everything else slowly falls into place.

Measuring the Chasm

You may be blessed with a totally understanding family and set of saintly friends for whom your illness poses no emotional challenges. More likely, however, your family and friends are human beings subject to the same confusion, petty jealousies and denial that you are dealing with.

Let's look at a few of the problems that can result when someone asks a person with chronic illness, "How are you?" If you're the patient, you may desperately want others to understand and appreciate your difficult situation. But deciding "how you are" at times may be so complicated, involving so many bodily functions, that you might wish you could hand out a reading from some kind of computer rather than explain it all. And if you've lived with chronic illness for a long time, you know that sometimes "how you are" may be determined only in retrospect.

In fact, you may have been through all this so many times that you've simply clammed up, because talking candidly about your condition is so painful and sticky. Perhaps you've hidden your illness out of embarrassment or self-consciousness. Or maybe you just get sick and tired of saying you're sick and tired.

Of course, the person asking the question may not really want to know "how you are." He or she may not care about your complex physical infirmities. The question may be simply a social inquiry, a way of beginning a conversation – or a ploy to get you to ask the same question in return.

People who deal with chronic illness every day speak a different language from those who don't. Both may use the same words, but attach entirely different meanings to them. "Illness" to the healthy may mean acute problems lasting a few days, weeks or even months, with medications that will soon clear everything up.

"Illness" for the incurably, chronically sick means a lifetime of days filled with ongoing, fluctuating health problems that have no easy solutions or quick answers. Most healthy people think there are two outcomes to illness: You either get well or you die. Few understand the concept of getting sick, staying sick and never really feeling well.

Our culture values quick solutions with visible results. Unsolvable problems, such as chronic illness, may be viewed as failures. From all the commercials on television, you would think that surely there's a pill for every ache and a cure for every problem?! You may find some people become frustrated if, over time, your response to "How are you?" doesn't report improvement.

Most healthy people have to experience months with a chronically ill loved one to move beyond a surface understanding of the condition. Even at that, the understanding will be limited. Until those who aren't ill walk a mile in your shoes, *they just don't and can't get it*, and they don't know that they don't get it! Both parties need to realize the dimensions of the chasm before they can bridge it.

Whether you're sick or well, only a precious few can share the depths of your soul and circumstances. That's the nature of life and the human heart. Identifying these special support persons and recruiting their help is especially crucial for you as a person with a chronic illness. Finding just a few who care can lessen the sting of what may seem to be indifference or avoidance from many others.

Another thorny issue is that your significant others may be constantly asked how you are doing. People may never think to ask how they are doing.

You Look Mahvelous!

Even after years of chronic illness, you may still look great. Of course, that can be both a blessing and a curse. Your healthy appearance may lead others – or you – to doubt how sick you really are. The old saying, "If you look good, you'll feel good," isn't true for everyone. You may look great but really feel lousy! Others, however, may assume your appearance is a true reflection of your physical state.

Often, when I answered, "How are you?" truthfully, telling people about my physical problems, their response was, "But you look so good!" I never got so many compliments on how good I looked until I became ill. You'd have thought I'd won a beauty queen title instead of a diagnosis! I began to view these "compliments" suspiciously. They started to feel like a put-down or denial of my situation.

Some people simply refused to believe I was sick, no matter how hard I tried to explain it, because I "looked so good!" to them. Eventually, I learned to save my breath. I knew I was sick – if they wouldn't or couldn't accept that fact, it wasn't really my problem.

The sanctioned "sick role" usually expects you to be dependent, childlike and whining, but especially to look sick. When living with chronic illness, you can't constantly act out the sick role and be emotionally healthy.

After a few such encounters, however, you may be torn between covering the illness' effects with makeup and looking the best you can, or allowing the effects of your illness to be visible, unquestionable and undeniable to everyone you meet.

Always projecting your illness with your external image can lead to other problems. Appearances are important in our culture, and wearing the prevailing identity of "I am illness" makes it difficult for you to relate to others from your former life. This may result in further losses of relationships and more grief.

How you look may not relate to your physical state, but your appearance can correspond to your emotional state. Learning to separate how you feel physically from how you feel emotionally will allow you to discuss your condition honestly and openly.

In trying to lift your spirits emotionally by looking your best, you may not look sick. During those times, it may be hard for others to understand that you don't feel well. Sometimes, you'll need to "own" your illness and neither cover up nor exaggerate it. Some of these occasions might be when you see the doctor, when you're in the hospital, when you're around understanding friends and family, or during times of increased disease activity, when you are forced to depend on others to carry out your daily duties.

Other times, it may be appropriate to play down your illness, but not in a way that denies it. Those occasions might be when you're at work, or meeting new friends, or going out for a special occasion. Constantly trying to "pass" for something that you aren't, however, creates a lot of stress, tension and anxiety.

It may take some time to know where, when and with whom you can own your illness, and how much of it to share, when greeted with the question, "How are you?" You'll goof up sometimes – be easy on yourself when you do.

Part of how you feel about yourself involves your sexuality. Awareness of your sexual identity so penetrates the fabric of adult life that you lose any consciousness of its presence until it is threatened or overshadowed by a new reality, such as a diagnosis of chronic illness. Such labels can displace your sexual identity as male or female, so that you begin to think of yourself as "a person with arthritis" or "a diabetic" or "a cancer patient" rather than as a man or a woman.

Hold on to all you can from your healthy life. That includes your good looks, your sexuality, your sense of humor, your faith and your matchless fashion sense. Whether your looks become a blessing or a curse is all in the way you handle it. You don't always need to identify yourself only with your illness. Remember your total identity as a person, accentuating the positive. You can be the best-looking, sexy sick person there ever was!

The Answer Is ...

Still, you may suffer anger, bitterness and a sense of isolation – even from a simple question like "How are you?" – until both sides understand these brief exchanges better. It may take a while to become comfortable with yourself and others in these moments.

In the meantime, you're still in the quandary of knowing how to respond. Sometimes, the less said, the better – a short bulletin about your condition may be more effective than a documentary to let people know that you don't need them to hover over you. As a rule, answering: "I'm okay ... fair ... making it" may suffice, and allow the inquirer to seek his or her own level of interest.

If you want to give some indication of difficulties without going into details, you can use such replies as: "I've been better and I've been worse." "Fair, some good and some bad." "I'm hanging in there." "I'm keeping my head above water."

Probe the situation directly with someone you know well by jokingly asking, "Do you want a lie, or do you want the truth?" Humor puts you and others at ease and your circumstances in perspective.

Some comebacks to "But you look so good!" might be:

"Well, I really work at it." "War paint can work wonders." "Thank goodness, all that beauty rest does some good." "You look pretty good yourself," or just a simple "Thank you!" Enjoy a compliment when it's given.

When you're confronted with someone who doesn't want to accept your condition, you'll never get anywhere trying to prove that looks don't give the whole story. Save yourself some energy – don't enter into this power struggle.

Understanding some of the dynamics of the question, "How are you?" allows you to relax when you answer. As you become more comfortable with yourself and your illness, others will be more at ease as well. Don't give up. There are those precious few out there who can share your journey. It may take a lot of faith and perseverance to find them.

In the meantime, here are a few responses to try:

. . . "I may look like a million, but I feel like a plug nickel."
. . . "It's a daily crap shoot."
. . . "It's a daily experiment."
. . . "On a scale of 1 to 10, I'm a 5."
. . . "The mind is fine, but the body is a sick joke."
. . . "I've had a pretty good week, but today I'm struggling."

And don't forget to ask, "And how are things going with you?"

---

1. Write down some automatic responses that might work for you.
2. List ways you handle the topic of disability with other people.
3. Using how you emotionally respond to the question "How are you?" as a barometer of your level of acceptance, how are you doing?

CHAPTER 13

Relationships and Support

The Relationship Dance

Life changes like illness and divorce may dramatically alter your emotional support systems. Some may strengthen, becoming deeper and more meaningful than ever. Others you'd counted on in the past may slowly and silently pull away. You may also find new support in unexpected places.

People with chronic illness sustain many devastating losses. Some important losses are body image, privacy and human relationships. The strong, supportive relationships that helped you through the diagnosis or a crisis may taper off just as you're fully coming to grips with the reality of your situation, two or three months down the road. The loss of these relationships may sting and be very painful and difficult to handle.

Friends and relatives may be affected by your illness in peculiar ways. Don't take their reactions personally. Their responses may have more to do with their own problems and fears than with you.

The able-bodied may grow weary and possibly disillusioned by the ill person's inability to return to their world of involvement and independence. Some may become angry when the ill person "refuses" to come home or return to work where he belongs.

Others may be frightened by illness or, in fact, anyone who is different from them. Your problems may be a threatening reminder of their own vulnerabilities. Denying their own human frailties, they must also deny them in you. These people will tend to avoid you because your very existence demands them to face and understand more than they can handle.

Close friends may become overloaded with feelings, and ignore you. Some may become stoic, suggest the latest remedy, or spout positive platitudes. Others may feel awkward and at a loss for words. Still others may become overly concerned, swoop down and try to "fix" you. Such "rescuers" often invade your boundaries in the process.

When you fall ill and stay ill, those around you may feel sorry for you or experience survivor's guilt. The more they feel sorry for you, the more vulnerable and threatened they may feel by what's happened to you. Pity is unhealthy for all involved.

You may be placed on a pedestal for your "wonderful attitude" of merely living and being ill. Really, you're just an average Joe, making it the best you can with the cards life has dealt you – just like everyone else.

At the same time, you may increase your own isolation because you are confused and uncomfortable with yourself: You withdraw as others pull away.

Consciously or unconsciously, you may also victimize loved ones as you withdraw or attack in confusion or anger. No one really goes through a problem alone. You take bystanders with you. You may not intend to hurt anyone, but under stress, your normal human reactions can be pretty ugly. Acting defensively, you may fail to see the wreckage around you.

You'll need to learn some new steps in this elaborate relationship dance. It's important not to withdraw: Research shows that people live longer, and have a better quality of life, with and without physical problems, if they join support groups and stay connected with life. Studies have shown a connection between talking about problems and a strengthened immune system, as well as other beneficial physical and psychological effects. Part of trauma resolution therapy revolves around the theory that talking about a problem actually changes your brain chemistry, reorganizes your thinking and shrinks a problem down to size. Trauma resolution therapy lists diagnosis of a chronic illness alongside traumas such as a natural disaster or a physical attack.

Help Wanted: Support Person

Be prepared to find support in surprising places. Casual friends, sensitized by events in their own lives, may come forward to sustain you. Often, your best support people will have been touched by grief themselves – they've "been there."

You may also find that you can affect how others relate to you, according to the image you project. If you act like a sick, dependent person, that's how you'll be treated. But if you want to be treated like an independent human being who's still responsible for yourself, act like one.

Until you are comfortable with yourself, others can't be comfortable with you. It may take some education, self-examination and counseling to help you get there.

At one point, I realized I was putting people in a double-bind. I wanted them to acknowledge my illness and daily struggle, but not treat me any differently from anyone else. Yikes!

Eventually, a few precious supportive relationships will emerge. It may take time and a lot of patience to discover these people, but they will slowly become apparent. They will simply be there with you to share your hurts and pains or joys and victories. Often, it may be up to you to take the first step toward finding support, because people may not know how to react to you.

Experiencing grief or illness isn't an absolute prerequisite to becoming a good support person, but it helps. A sensitive, caring soul who knows your background can also join the ranks of the few. In reaching out to lend support to someone else, you may also find support for yourself.

Through trial and error, you may establish a grading process of receptivity levels of the people around you. Grade Ones can hear the whole story without trying to "fix" you. Grade Twos can hear only a condensed version. Grade Threes only want an "I'm OK" or "I'm not so good." Grade Fours want to hear only "Everything is fine." This ranking may take some time, and people may shift back and forth between grades, depending on what's happening in their lives.

Spread It Around

Once you've found a support person, keep in mind that he or she may not be around forever or all of the time. Interests shift, lives take different directions and contact may be lost. Some will hang in there. Others won't.

Your spouse or family members may not be able to support you at all or may be supportive only at times. If they can't be supportive, they can't. Accept them as they are. You can't force them to be something they're unable to be. They need support themselves.

Look elsewhere and spread out a broad base of support among several people, maybe including a counselor so you can maintain balance. The martial arts show that you can withstand a blow better and not loose your balance if your weight is spread over a broad base of support. Put one foot in front of the other and spread your feet apart.

At a time of diagnosis or crisis, you may need to talk incessantly about the illness and yourself. This need lessens with time, as the illness becomes an integrated part of your life rather than your main focus, and support lines are identified.

Your family may grow understandably weary during these times and may require more help than usual themselves. They are juggling their own fears and uncertainties in addition to yours, while trying to maintain balance. They may fear failure. Don't forget to encourage, thank and help them whenever you can.

Make your support system a two-way street. Remember that even those closest to you may need a vacation from sharing problems when grappling with difficulties of their own. Respect their privacy, limitations and schedules.

Taking Charge

When you are hurting, you can suffer in an irresponsible, manipulative way. Complaining, making others feel guilty, placing excessive demands on your friends, and expecting people to do what you can do by yourself leads to a helpless, self-pitying attitude. By shifting blame onto others, you have found a way to avoid doing something about your own problems.

Ultimately, you alone are responsible for taking care of yourself: physically, emotionally, mentally and spiritually. *No one* can do it for you. Others can only encourage you and offer advice. Your doctor, psychiatrist, pastor, family and friends are only guides and supports. You need to do the real work yourself.

Assuming responsibility for yourself is the first step toward emotional, physical and spiritual health. The second step is realizing you need to take care of yourself first before you can take care of anyone else. Any other commitments rank second or you will shortchange all involved – mainly you! Education and counseling can help you sort out priorities if you have problems with putting your own care first.

Your chronic illness affects each individual member of your family and the unit's functioning as a whole. Avoid becoming a passive victim or an aggressive manipulator who complicates your already difficult situation. Instead, resolve to find healthy ways to cooperate with those around you. You may withdraw into you own world of self-pity, helplessness and bitterness without the objectivity, support and encouragement of those who care.

As time passes, you'll find your support network. Those precious ones who are able to go the distance with you will become rare treasures. The real wealth of this life is to be found in those relationships. Initiating and nurturing these ties may become your new, No. 1 priority – a reward for being forced to slow down and appreciate what's around you.

A joy shared is multiplied. A burden shared is divided!

CHAPTER 14

It's a Family Affair

All for One ...

Adjustment to a chronic illness is a family affair. You may think of it as "your illness," but the stresses affect everyone around you. Chronic illness involves a sequence of phases, including diagnosis, flares, remission and, finally, death, that the family best addresses as a group. Failure to cope with one phase may derail coping for the next phase, and thereby the entire process.

Your family's reaction to your illness can greatly affect your own adjustment to it. If you can anticipate being included as part of the functioning family unit, with as many of your former roles preserved as possible to accommodate your limitations, you are more likely to actively participate in your treatment program.

Family rules and roles, many of them unconscious, may need to be consciously modified along new priorities, as ongoing illness becomes a part of your daily lives.

Starting from Scratch

Handling any crisis successfully requires comprehending (even hazily) what the crisis means to everyday living and future plans; minimizing the time it takes to face the painful circumstances; and getting on with life as it exists in the present. If the family can mourn the loss of life as it used to be together, each can find comfort and solace in one another. Mourning may take a long time or can seem to be brief, only to resurface intermittently.

The first task is to squarely face the diagnosis and what it means. You or other family members may go into denial, expressed by flights of activity, such as changing jobs or moving, shopping for a cure, or spending money unnecessarily. These evasive maneuvers only add to the burden to be carried by all.

Family members may disagree on how to define the illness, with whom to discuss it, and what to tell others about it. If everyone doesn't pitch in to help meet new responsibilities, resentment may brew. The joint effort essential for family coping and functioning may be further damaged.

Not every family member will join the effort. More distant family members, such as grandparents, grandchildren, cousins, aunts and uncles, may not know how to help. Even close family members, including siblings or spouses, may be unable or unwilling to pitch in.

Crisis has a way of stirring the emotional pot and bringing everything to the surface. Longstanding, unspoken jealousies and power struggles that have simmered quietly beneath the family dynamic may erupt into a full-blown family feud as you are diagnosed with a significant health problem.

In the long run, in fact, some families may be more hurtful than helpful until adjustments are made. Once the old family structure shatters, old roles die, shift and are reconstructed. Some family members may want to fight these necessary adjustments, and try to revert to the familiar steps of the old family dance before you became ill. You may not be able to fulfill those old roles.

Families need to find new ways to play together. Your old recreations – hiking, camping, tennis, etc.– may be lost and need to be creatively replaced. New ways of playing together can be found: putting together jigsaw puzzles, renting videos, playing board games.

Ultimately, healthier patterns of behavior and relating may emerge. Family members who are able to take your lead and dance to this new tune may bond closer than ever. But some families may eventually fall apart. It all depends on each person staying self-focused to learn all they can about themselves, rather than trying to change others in the family.

If your marriage or family relationships were already troubled before you became ill, the challenges will most likely escalate with the additional stress of medical problems. You will need to begin to deal with the difficulties within your family before you can successfully deal with the challenges of chronic illness.

Stress may escalate to its highest level when you reach a plateau with your illness. You and your family may realize this is as good as it is going to get – what it's going to be like for all of you the rest of your life. Such a realization can fuse a family together in an uncomfortable mesh of emotions.

Keep the lines of communication open with gut-level honesty. Freely express anger, hurt, frustration, joy and laughter about what's happening. The family that cries, yells, plays and laughs together may stay together! You need to share it all.

Accepting others' differing ways of handling problems may open the door to new ways of coping together.

Some families may require outside help to work out their problems. Don't be afraid to admit that you or your family may benefit from guidance. Family therapy, group counseling or individual counseling can help point out blind spots so you can face and celebrate life with chronic illness together.

Family Roles and Codependence

I found that stepping into my new life took more than time. My loved ones needed to formulate new roles and rules for living together. Unconscious family "scripts" that had been passed on for generations – with their unwritten expectations of roles and dialogues concerning secrecy, boundaries and self-expression – needed to be rewritten.

No matter how healthy or wonderful your family of origin, you probably were emotionally wounded to some degree in childhood. There's no way any parent can completely meet a child's needs. Perhaps your father was domineering and controlling. Or your mother left the family, and you will always fear abandonment. The scars may have formed from less dramatic injuries – perhaps a parent was unavailable emotionally, too busy from work or caring for other family members. Perhaps he or she was too strict or intrusive. We're all humans and we all err.

Even in "perfect" families, your childhood hurts influenced your personality development. To take care of your emotional wounds and survive in your family of origin, you adopted a lifestyle and personality to cope. (You'll learn more about this in Chapters 22 and 23 – "Lifestyle Engineering" and "Personality Engineering.")

Your childhood choice of how you learned to interface with

your world may have worked well in your family of origin but may not be healthy for you now in a different time and setting. Your defense mechanisms that worked before may not work in a healthy way with those around you now. The only way I knew to get what I needed or set my boundaries was to get sick. The personality I developed to cope with my childhood put the care of others before my own needs, and I ignored my own health problems until they became severe.

One strategy for understanding relationships is Imago theory (the name combines the words "image" and "ego"). This philosophy states that you are attracted to people who were wounded at the same stage and age that you were as a child. Your partner and friends may have found an opposite way from you to take care of themselves. In this attraction process you unconsciously bring to yourself parts of yourself that you have rejected, suppressed or denied. The whole unconscious effort of coupling is to complete yourself.

Unless you work on making the attraction process conscious, the person or people you are attracted to – including your mate – may end up wounding you all over again, in the same way you were hurt as a child. This happens more often in times of extreme stress such as living with chronic illness. Stress can make behaviors become unhealthy and lifestyles more rigid and fixed.

Whether or not your emotional wounds ever heal depends on your making conscious the effects of the problematic relationships that hurt you in childhood. Seeing how I continue to play out my emotional wounds with people in the present helps me make healthy conscious choices from my head and heart instead of unhealthy reactions from my gut.

When illness strikes, you may not have the luxury of continuing familiar, but emotionally destructive relationships. Your diminished stamina may limit the amount of time you can spend fixing or maintaining them. A decision to mend or end energy-consuming and emotionally painful relationships really may be a choice between life and death for you. I feel that I *chose life* for myself by growing, acknowledging and working through some of the emotional wounds that were rooted in my childhood. However, the choices I made upset the fit and balance of my marriage and led to divorce.

Unhealthy and dysfunctional patterns of relating can become even more problematic in times of stress, such as when you're ill. One such pattern that was particularly troublesome in my family was codependence.

Codependence involves two people who consistently play out the roles of victim and caretaker. A spouse (or even a health-care worker) who hovers, always ready to rush to the rescue at the smallest sign of trouble, may encourage the chronically ill person to assume the role of victim. Such caretakers may enjoy rescuing so much that deep down, they don't really wish the victim to get better. The thought of the victim not needing their help may be threatening.

On the other hand, a chronically ill spouse may find it impossible to continue his or her role as rescuer. This happened in my marriage and many of my other relationships. I'd always been there to take care of Jim emotionally. After I fell ill, however, I physically couldn't keep up many of the roles I'd assumed, including that of my husband's rescuer. If a relationship cannot grow past the need for victims and rescuers, it may not survive.

In the long run, both people in a codependent relationship become victims. The caretaker may try to read the victim's mind, to intuit what the victim wants or needs, only to be greeted with indifference or hostility from the victim.

Rebalancing codependency means becoming interdependent and using "I" statements to set your boundaries clearly and to ask for what you need. Such statements as "I can dress myself, thank you," or "I need help with sorting the laundry today" put yourself in charge. Avoid using "you" statements, which often imply blame, as in "You don't need to button my shirt," or "You never help me with the laundry." Such statements also head off the need for a mind-reading caretaker.

The bony, pointing finger of blame and shame in "you" statements is destructive for all involved. You give away all of your power with "you" statements. You only have the power to change yourself. You need to move from using should, out, must, have to, got to … "musturbating" to needs, wants, likes, thinks, feels.

RX for Counseling

Perhaps you've tried the same old thing over and over again to solve family problems. Try some new solutions – the old ones actually can become the problem! A marriage or family therapist is trained to look at your family and help find new and healthier ways of functioning and communicating. It's very difficult to get well in the midst of an unhealthy family.

To learn more about Imago therapy, you may want to read Harville Hendrix's books, *Getting the Love You Want* and *Keeping the Love You Find*. Imago therapy gives a framework to understand what happens in the attraction process and marriage. Imago books, tapes and workshops also teach communication skills that break the cycle of repeated wounding and allow healing. For more information call 1-800-729-1121.

CHAPTER 15

You and Your Doctor

I have a surgeon friend who greets each new cancer patient with, "You and I are getting married! We're going to be in this together for a long time – maybe the rest of your life. I'll be honest with you and I want you to be honest with me. If you don't like something or you disagree with me, please tell me. We'll work it out."

The doctor-patient relationship really is a marriage for the chronically ill – it's one of the most important bonds in their lives. There will be give-and-take, agreements and disagreements. It is a relationship best maintained with honesty, concern and respect by both parties. No doctor is perfect, as no patient is perfect. And as in a marriage, personalities need to naturally blend to some degree.

Just as marriages often take place in the heat of passion – perhaps not the best way to choose a partner for life – you may need to find a doctor when you're at your lowest physical or emotional point. Only time will tell if your partnership will be sound. The relationship will be long-term, with the doctor's opinions and judgments reaching into many areas and decisions of your life.

For wedded bliss between you and your physician, you'll want a balanced, working partnership. But just as in marriage, doctor-patient interactions can be affected by all-too-human emotions. You may displace your anger about the illness and loss of privacy on the doctor, since there may be no other acceptable target for these feelings. The doctor may also displace feelings of frustration on you.

A power struggle may develop to establish who's in charge. The doctor, who may be used to wielding a great deal of power, may find it difficult to relinquish some control to you, and vice versa. What may be for the doctor just another fleeting moment in a long day of many patients may be for you a long-awaited and remembered "holy moment," to be played and replayed many times in your mind.

During this "holy moment," the whole direction of your life may be changed. Your suspected diagnosis may be officially confirmed. Your diet, functions or mobility may be restricted. Scary questions may be answered, leading to scarier questions.

Meanwhile, your anxiety may be so heightened that you can't hear a thing, much less understand complex medical terminology. Your mind may go into orbit, not to return to earth for some time. You may need to go over and over the same material with the doctor on return visits, in order to absorb it all.

Like all humans involved in a relationship, you and your doctor may project your own emotions, motivations and behaviors on each other. Patients looking for authority may see the doctor as a father figure. Patients may fall in love, in a sense, with their doctors. Each may seek approval and affirmation from the other.

Sexuality plays an important part in all relationships, and the doctor-patient relationship is no exception. Over the years, the doctor will be involved in and acquainted with just about every intimate detail of your life, from your sleep patterns to your libido.

The intimacy of your relationship may lead you to want a closer, more personal connection with your doctor. The doctor may need his or her professional distance. At times, too, health-care professionals overstep boundaries: I have seen codependent relationships in which doctors who envision themselves as supreme rescuers cripple patients who view themselves as victims.

Your doctor is subject to the same emotions you're struggling with. Medical professionals perform under the continual pressure of making rapid life-or-death decisions, running an office, and dealing with the restrictions and mandates of managed care.

Physicians' training emphasizes relieving pain and suffering rather than helping people learn how to live with it. Your chronic distress may present him or her with personal distress.

Doctors aren't gods – they're just as human as you are. Their lives may be no better integrated than the patients they try to treat or sustain.

The medical arena can be emotionally charged. Anger and hurt – sometimes justified, sometimes not – needs to be addressed and appropriately vented. However, if your vigorous communication efforts fail, sometimes the only healthy answer for a troubled "marriage" with your doctor is divorce.

Think carefully about a decision to change doctors. It may take months or years to cultivate a new relationship. Real-life events shared by a doctor and patient are difficult to duplicate in a written or verbal report. A new doctor may start all over again, questioning or rejecting your diagnosis and treatment.

The best doctor-patient relationships balance dependence and independence. Assume responsibility for your life in all arenas (mind, body, spirit, family, society) and negotiate the business of managing your health. No doctor can keep you in good health. He or she can only offer guidance, support and encouragement. You do the hard work! Your doctor will give you some information about your illness, but your body will also tell you what's going on. Compare the two interpretations. From this input, you formulate a plan of action.

Your doctor needs to allow you, as an equal partner, to assume an active role in your treatment as you take responsibility for yourself. The healthy evolution of this partnership depends on trust, honesty, respect, caring and commitment from both parties.

PART III

Learning the
Medical Ropes

CHAPTER 16

"What's Up, Doc?"

Oops! I forgot to ask my doctor about that medicine. By golly, I failed to tell him about my rash! My mind gets so boggled and I get so tongue-tied at doctor's visits! I can't remember when something started, or how!" Does this ever happen to you?

In the first stages after my diagnosis, I would come away from my doctor's appointments totally frustrated. There would be so much happening between visits that I would want to get a reading on from my doctor.

Without fail, I would forget something really important or go completely blank in the emotionally heightened atmosphere of the doctor's office. This would result in frustration and unresolved anxiety. Over the years, I developed a system that has helped me communicate with my doctors, who have most graciously adapted to my idiosyncratic methods.

Your doctor's visits are important business meetings, and you should make the best use of your time. So try to come up with a professional, businesslike approach for preparing for and conducting these meetings.

Between visits, I keep a running diary of occurrences that I want to tell my doctor about. Using a regular month-at-a glance calendar is a good way to keep track of your schedule, watch for symptom patterns, and figure out cause-and-effect.

If you prefer, you can keep track instead on a homemade month-at-a-glance grid on a legal pad. I put the date down the side and my unique symptoms across the top. I rate the symptoms mild (#1) with black ink, moderate (#2) in blue ink, severe (#3) in red ink. I really can see where and how depression, loss of sleep or increased activity escalate pain or fatigue.

I also jot down questions that come to mind. Writing down even the most minor and silly questions helps me get them off my mind. It also helps me become acquainted with my individual illness patterns in response to my life, emotions and schedules. A day or so before the visit, I go over my list of questions and observations.

I scratch off some questions that have been resolved on their own and or haven't proven to be significant. Sometimes I add others that occur to me while reading the list. Some details might not be of great significance in terms of altering treatment, but might give the doctor a picture of ongoing or declining disease activity. Other items might be of greater concern.

On my calendar I include physical symptoms, emotional state (if I'm having problems), appointments with other doctors, what other doctors have said at visits with me, information about work status or current activities, billing problems – anything that might give the doctor a complete picture of what is going on with me.

I type or write the information and questions on what I call my update list as neatly and concisely as possible, and keep a copy for myself. I prioritize my concerns and questions because I know my time with the doctor will be limited and we may not get to everything.

Writing everything down forces me to clarify my thinking. It's far easier to review my list than to try to verbalize everything in the doctor's office. The list is also particularly helpful when you're seeing several doctors. You have a way of checking what you have mentioned to which doctor, and when.

At my visit, I give my doctor his copy of my list, questions and present concerns to keep in my chart. This allows him to scan what I have put down, commenting on items he feels are significant and need follow-up, and passing over less important items. If he doesn't pick up on something I'm particularly concerned about, I ask him about it.

Focusing on the most important points allows me more time to discuss them. The doctor may reinforce information I'd forgotten, or that he hadn't clearly communicated. I keep my copies, update them with test results and answers to questions, and file them.

SAMPLE UPDATE

Dr. Tom Jones- 7/3/99
Update
1. pain - having pain in
        - hand
        - hip
        - knee
        - chest wall
        - neck

2. fatigue - not able to be functional but a few hours a day
3. fever - runs from 99.4 to 100.2 each day

Questions-
1. What I do about my prednisone dose – now 15 mg a day?
2. What did my last labs show about my disease activity? May I have a copy?

My system has come to serve as a diary that gives me feedback on response to medications as well as illness fluctuations as related to other parts of my life. It also helps me observe disease activity and patterns in relation to seasonal changes and activities.

In addition to serving as my personal diary, it can also serve as a source of valuable documentation if needed for insurance or disability purposes. It is difficult to rely just on memory for certain dates or events. Using this approach has helped on many levels.

I still forget things and end up calling, faxing or writing my doctor! Even so, I usually feel we've covered a lot of ground during a visit. From my doctor's response I can pick up on which things to just add to the "live with it" list while keeping an eye on them as an indication of disease activity, and which things might need more attention with additional follow-up.

Try this process yourself, adapting it with your own variations and ideas. It may work for you and your doctor and it may not. Its purpose is to make the best use possible of the short time you have with your doctor, and to make the visits less stressful.

As a side benefit, two-way communication between you may improve. Remember, your doctor is not the boss at these business meetings. You're partners, and it's up to you to make sure you're doing your part.

CHAPTER 17

Going to the Hospital

As you probably already know, if you have a chronic illness, you may to need to go to the hospital from time to time. Whether it's because of acute exacerbations of the illness or for re-evaluations, diagnostic work or corrective surgery, you're probably not going to look forward to it with great joy.

Hospitalizations may make those around you suddenly more aware of your illness, even if the problems have been there all along. You may get a lot of extra attention, and your forces may rally to bring in food, take charge of the house and hover over your children, which may embarrass them to death. Teenagers, especially, may want to shrink into the woodwork. Let them know that you're aware this experience is trying for them too, and allow them time to be with their friends.

You may find that going into the hospital bolsters your credibility of being sick with family, friends, health-care professionals or insurance providers. It's difficult for most people to realize that you can be ill while remaining functional and even cheerful. A hospital stay may force them to acknowledge you're really dealing with a serious illness. That may be stressful to you both, but in the long run, it may also be beneficial.

You and your family's emotional, physical and financial resources may be drained as hospitalizations turn family routines, schedules and budgets into chaos. All may be strained to meet the increased demands.

Creating an emergency plan with everyone who'll be involved can be helpful, especially in emergency situations. Writing all the pertinent information down and leaving it in a central place can be helpful for everyone.

I have an emergency plan on the bulletin board next to the phone in my kitchen. I've included insurance information; important phone numbers including the doctor, pharmacy and vet; my list of medications; how to water the plants; etc. I try to consider anything that will need to be done in my absence. If you decide to write up such a plan, try to imagine what people would need to know to keep your household running in your absence.

If visits or phone calls from friends and family just add to the strain, be honest. Tell your support community what you and your family do and don't need to help you through this difficult time.

After you've been hospitalized repeatedly, these events may become old hat to your family and friends. They may remain a big deal to you! Let your support units know.

Before You Go:
Negotiating the Details

Before a couple of my many surgeries during and after my divorce, my teenaged sons, Jamie and Keith, and I went to see the family therapist to negotiate my needs. I let them know that this was A BIG DEAL for me and I needed their support and help! They set boundaries on what they could and couldn't do for me.

They let me know that putting the whole community on alert about my illness embarrassed them. As teenagers, they were acutely and uncomfortably aware of being made to feel different from everybody else. At their ages, they most wanted just to blend in with everybody else. They also felt that certain people in our support community treated them like children and invaded our family boundaries too much.

However, as a single parent, I had certain responsibilities: I wanted to be sure the boys would never be alone in the house; that they were always to let me know where they were; and that they were to keep their same curfews. I recruited trusted friends and neighbors to help.

We even negotiated food needs. The boys felt if we bought a loaf of bread and a jar of peanut butter that we'd do just fine! I didn't buy their plan. We bartered on who would be asked to bring in food and what to tell them to bring. Yucky vegetable casseroles were banned.

The boys let me know who they were comfortable with coming to stay with them. They were at an age where they only needed someone to check in with and serve as a home base.

Over the years, I found several people who'd come and stay at the house in my absence. My goal, with the help of my counselor, was to provide a balance of freedom and structure appropriate to the boys' ages whether I was in the hospital or not.

Jamie and Keith couldn't bear to visit me in the hospital. That would be the ultimate admission that their dad had left us and they were filling his role. They would call and check in on me. When I got home I knew to expect not TLC, but LLC (loud loving care).

I was determined not to cast the boys into any adult roles or expect them to fill duties their dad or other absent family members did not fill. I didn't want adult roles thrust on them as they had been on me growing up.

My counselor, the boys and I negotiated that I would maintain expectations realistic to their ages and their activities would be as undisturbed as possible. Jamie and Keith did find their own ways to be attentive and caring that really touched me. I relied on my counselor and family of friends to fill any adult roles needed.

Putting too much responsibility on teenagers of parents with illness, especially compounded by divorce, can interrupt their launching into their own lives. They may need to totally run away, act out in order to leave the home, or they may stay home and be rescuers. My boys seem to have launched pretty well, given all they had to go through in growing up.

Your children may wish to visit you in the hospital. If you would find that comforting, perhaps one of your support people could take them, and try to make it as unscary as possible. Explaining what the medical equipment is for and letting them see where you are may be comforting.

Realistic expectations of what we could expect of each other made hospitalizations, which could have been devastating, a growing experience in how to negotiate with each other. With the help of the counselor, we assertively, clearly and directly set our boundaries and asked for what we needed with "I" messages. WOW! What a difference!

Hospitality

Hospital procedures can be more unbearable than the condition that sent you there. Here are a few tips on how to make it through a hospital stay.

1. The medical directive NPO (an abbreviation for the Latin *non per os*; nothing by mouth) is often given for 12 hours before a lab test or procedure. It presents special problems for patients with a dry mouth or Sjögren's syndrome. Here are a few tricks:
   - rinse mouth out with mouthwash or brush teeth, being careful not to swallow
   - suck a slightly damp washrag, letting dry mucous membranes absorb the moisture
   - apply lip balm
   - drink plenty of fluids right up to the time for NPO to begin
   - ask for a vaporizer
   - ask if you can be allowed to chew gum.

2. In prolonged visits, hospital sheets may rub your elbows raw. Putting alcohol on your elbows at the beginning of a stay to dry them out will make them tougher, and the sheets won't rub as much.

3. To ease nausea:
   - eat small, frequent meals
   - breathe deeply, from your abdomen
   - suck on ice chips
   - drink carbonated beverages or hot tea
   - apply a cold compress to your forehead

- eat dry toast or crackers
- make sure the room is cool

4. Bring extra pillows from home to help position painful joints. When lying on your side, a pillow between the knees can prevent hip rotation. Use a pillow to support your arm and shoulder.

5. Change bed position frequently to help alleviate back discomfort, sore joints or difficulty breathing. If you're having trouble breathing, position the hospital bed so your head is up over halfway, and the knees elevated.

6. Cheese crackers, if permitted in your diet, help take away the bad taste of medications.

7. Use cotton balls or earplugs to shut out hospital or roommate's noises so you can sleep.

8. Dry hospital heat can dry out your sinuses. A vaporizer provides moisture and white noise to drown out other sounds.

9. When pain or discomfort is intense, you'll be able to bear it better if you practice visualizing beautiful scenery or pleasant memories.

10. Isometric exercises (tightening and relaxing muscle groups), wiggling toes, flexing muscles and deep breathing exercises (even while confined to bed) can help promote relaxation and increase circulation.

11. Some hospital procedures require lying still in uncomfortable positions for long periods of time. Try:
    • focusing on points in the room to provide a diversion
    • wiggling toes or any part of the body in a rotating manner
    • or anything that would help you focus away from lying still.

12. Whether or not you have circulation problems (such as Raynaud's phenomenon) that leave you with cold hands and feet, take extra blankets and several pairs of socks. Layers work best. Hospital temperatures can be cool. Emergency and operating rooms will actually heat blankets for you.

13. Remember to take your journal. Writing can pass time, as well as release anxiety about what you are going through.

In the age of managed care, hospitalizations are shorter and less frequent. Make the most of each stay. Once again, make it business, write down your observations and questions, and remember you're the one who is ultimately responsible for you.

CHAPTER 18

Medical Word Games

Words have no meaning except in the way you interpret them from your own experience. The same words may hold different meaning for you as your life unfolds and you experience their reality from different angles.

At one point in your life, a word may be connected with fear and depression. At another point, your reaction to the same word may be nonchalance. Only when your life translates a word into a living definition and experience do you fully understand its meaning. Until then, it remains just a word.

Medical personnel use words to describe, classify or categorize. These words, learned in training, may hold no meaning for them personally. Once applied to your condition, you may understand these terms in a way they never will.

As a nurse I had no idea what chronic illness and pain really meant. I'd only dealt with patients experiencing acute or terminal illness. Entering the ranks of the chronically ill certainly fleshed out my skeletal understanding of these terms. I began to formulate my own meanings of these words.

Unfamiliar words that never applied to you before may produce anxiety or pain. Educate yourself about them as you experience them to arrive at your own personal definition.

Let's review a few of them.

Mild/Severe

Illnesses may be medically categorized as "mild" or "severe." But there may be nothing mild about the illness to the person living with it. You may view a description of your condition as mild with mixed emotions, or as a slap in the face.

A condition that wreaks havoc on your life seems anything but mild. The classification seems to indicate that things should be "almost normal," or not awful, anyway. That's not always the case. For example, fatigue and sore muscles and joints may be more limiting than decreased kidney functioning.

In the medical sense, the word mild implies that the condition is not life threatening or has no serious long-term implications. The term gives no picture of your subjective experiences. You may find yourself thinking, "If this is mild, I'd hate to see what severe is!" Even though a mild condition may not result in death, you may feel like death warmed over.

When considering a condition such as systemic lupus erythematosus (SLE, an autoimmune collagen vascular disease), the patient with "mild" disease activity may experience fever, arthritis, inflammation of the lung and/or heart lining with small collections of fluid around either, fatigue and rash. Most people don't think of such symptoms as mild.

Severe, in medical terms, indicates a condition that may be

life-threatening or has serious long-term implications. Strange as it may seem, the person with severe disease activity may not feel as ill or be as incapacitated over long periods of time as the person with ongoing, mild problems. Mild disease isn't life-threatening, but it can be life-stifling.

The severely ill may justifiably warrant a lot of attention and empathy. Those categorized as mildly ill may find treatment delivered in a more lackadaisical manner. Interest of friends and family may come and go.

Although your disease may be categorized as mild, expensive lab tests may still need to be run on a regular basis as a matter of routine monitoring with no subsequent change in treatment or condition. Drug bills may sap your budget without providing any expectation that you're going to feel normal after taking them.

Ironically, severe illnesses may be relieved or cured with potent drugs or treatments. But in mild disease, many symptoms may have to be endured, since the risks of using toxic drugs is not warranted. You don't shoot a mosquito off your foot. The first watchword of the medical profession is "Do no harm."

Normal/Abnormal

Abnormal lab results or symptoms may produce an initial flurry of concern. As the months and years go by and disease activity establishes a pattern, the very same lab results may be accompanied with congratulations rather than concern. You are slowly establishing what is normal/abnormal and abnormal/abnormal for you, which may fluctuate over time.

Adapting to certain abnormal test results means living within different parameters, accepting tradeoffs and incorporating mild symptoms into your life, even though their consequences may not be mild. It also means learning to recognize when symptoms require further attention.

Acute/Chronic

Acute, although there is nothing cute about it, is defined medically as a condition usually having severe symptoms with a sudden onset and an expected short course.

The general public is more knowledgeable about this type of illness. You either improve and get well, or get worse, become terminal and die. The adrenaline pumps, quick solutions are aggressively sought and applied, and results are or aren't evident within a short time. An end is in sight.

Chronic is a condition that may persist for a long time with the possibility of fluctuating disease activity with little change in treatment. The pace of dealing with chronic illness needs to be slower and more flexible in order to prevent burnout for all involved. Chronic conditions are marathons; acute and terminal illnesses are sprints.

Chronic illness requires endurance. You may experience sprints of acute episodes or flares interspersed throughout the marathon. You'll need to switch your pace back and forth.

Strength and coping abilities may need to stretch out over long periods of time, with many bumps in the road. You may not get completely well or die, but learn to live with fluctuations in the ongoing illness. Your lifestyle may need to change in many ways, and continue to alter through the years.

Progressive/Phasic

Progressive illness is marked by continuous spreading or increasing severity with permanent accumulative damage and a downhill course. Progressive illnesses could lead to such serious outcomes as paralysis or death.

Phasic illnesses are distinguished by come-and-go flares seen in such illnesses as systemic lupus erythematosus (SLE), rheumatoid arthritis (RA) and multiple sclerosis (MS). A phasic illness involves erratic, unpredictable, up-and-down, back-and-forth motion with no clear course of illness, recovery and/or prognosis.

Disease/Illness

Now, here's a tricky one that really splits hairs. Illness and disease are not the same thing. A person may experience a series of symptoms and illnesses that when considered together fall under the umbrella of a disease. The symptoms or illnesses you manifest may include sore joints, fatigue, fever, weakness, muscle aches or pains, but your disease may be multiple sclerosis (MS), heart disease, diabetes, systemic lupus erythematosus (SLE), rheumatoid arthritis (RA) or cancer.

I had many illness episodes prior to the diagnosis of SLE: tendinitis, frequent infections, joint pain, severe toxemia with my second pregnancy. Each of these illness episodes stood alone until I earned the diagnosis of SLE that connected them all under the umbrella of one disease.

Many people may erroneously think that if a disease is identified, the progress of the illnesses you experience should be predictable. A diagnosis may put fragmented symptoms together into a completed puzzle, but in no way offers any magic control or treatment.

It's also helpful to realize that all illnesses you experience may not be parts of your diagnosed disease, but may stand alone or be related to something else entirely.

Curable/Incurable

A cure may be defined as the eradication of a disease. The slate is wiped clean of symptoms. Sometimes, months or years without symptoms may pass before a condition (such as cancer, for example) may be considered cured. On the other hand, a cure can come after just a 10-day course of antibiotics when you're treating a urinary tract infection.

Incurable may be defined as not susceptible to cure. It may imply that no cause has been discovered for the disease. You need to know what's broken and why before you can fix it. Similarly, the cause of a disease must be determined before a cure can be found. Knowing the cause, however, does not mean a cure is always available.

Chronic illness is often incurable. Usually, the symptoms are treated rather than the disease itself. The slate can't be wiped clean, but is kept as usable as possible.

As causes of more and more diseases are pinpointed, providing prevention or cure (for example, tuberculosis, smallpox, polio and cancer), hope and encouragement are offered to all. Research progress in one area may open doors to advances in others.

The Power of Words

Words are used to help frame an experience, and store it in your mind. Words that were once a big deal to you regarding your disease can become just the vocabulary you need to communicate about your illness. These words can become powerful tools to get the treatment you need, rather than sources of fear and anxiety.

CHAPTER 19

Pain

Is pain merely a signal that travels along nerves from the source of the pain to the brain and back? Why do some people have high pain tolerance and others low pain tolerance? Can your experience affect the way you perceive it?

Can pain be relieved by methods other than conventional medication and surgery? Can your mind's internal resources overcome pain?

By thinking of pain as more than merely the nerve connections to and from the brain, you can learn methods to help you cope with pain, and lessen its effects on your life.

Pain is a perceptual experience. That is, you first become aware of it through one of your senses, and then translate it into something meaningful: If you burn your hand on the stove, you feel the pain and jerk your hand away from the heat.

You learned how to respond to pain (your "pain behavior") in your family and culture. Pain behaviors learned in the family unit are tried out and reinforced or extinguished, maintained or adapted by your culture.

The quality and intensity of your pain is influenced by your unique past experience, by the meaning you assign to the cause of pain, and by your state of mind at the moment the pain is experienced.

You adapt more easily to pain when it is predictable and within control. Patients who are told beforehand what kind of pain to expect after surgery require less pain medication and recover more quickly than those who aren't informed.

Conversely, pain may worsen in an atmosphere of ambiguity. Fear and anxiety heighten pain, especially if it is interpreted as resulting from a life-threatening condition.

When your pain is associated with a beneficial outcome, such as childbirth or winning a game, it is not accompanied by anxiety. Suffering is then minimized or postponed. There are many stories of athletes with major injuries finishing a game or an event, only to collapse in pain afterwards.

Studies have also found that patients who communicate openly with their physicians require less pain medication, possibly because talking about pain may reduce anxiety. That release of psychological tension may account for why the patients felt less pain.

Pain often seems more intense when you are alone, at night, when you have no source of help or nothing to take your mind off it. Pain often worsens when the doctor is unavailable (like at night or during weekends) and when there is reduced outside stimulation to divert attention from it. Pain may astonishingly lessen once you're on your way to see the doctor.

High anxiety and depression reduce pain tolerance. Withdrawing into yourself and focusing solely on bodily functions will heighten your perception of pain. When your anxiety is low and you focus attention outward, rather than on your body, your pain tolerance is increased.

Some people tend to intensify their own pain. Others can reduce it. Lowering anxiety and staying in touch with the outside world seem to be key points in learning to lessen pain.

Anxiety may be reduced with understanding what the pain means and providing relief, whether by heat, traction, bracing, cold, massage, relaxation techniques, imagery, pain medication, exercise, rest, diversion, family and cultural dynamics, or your own unique personality and belief system.

Chronic pain lends itself more readily to adopting learned behaviors than does acute, short-lived pain. People's responses around you can either reinforce your pain behavior (by giving you more attention and thereby reducing anxiety), or negate pain behaviors. If your family coddles you constantly, you may find yourself wincing more or exaggerating your limp around them.

In a study of families dealing with chronic pain, patients' spouses were often lacking in resources to help them deal with the situation. These resources include spirituality, talking about their problems with others, or seeking information about the pain. Perhaps this happens in families because the person in pain becomes the main focus of the family. The well spouse may feel guilty thinking of him or herself when the loved one is ill.

Spouses who were highly stressed from other sources in their lives had the least resources to deal with their partner's pain. They handled the situation in a much more stressful manner for all concerned.

Roles that spouses assume in coping with chronic pain vary, but may include the protector-advocate (jumping to constantly protect and defend), the instructor-admonisher (lecturing and admonishing their partner on what to do and not to do), and the avoider-ignorer (sidestepping it all).

The protector role, involving many maneuvers on behalf of the spouse to insulate the partner in chronic pain, was found to be the most depleting approach. Once the spouse's resources are exhausted, his or her view of reality may become threatened. Fear or hopelessness may result. Combining or shifting among all the roles may be the most realistic approach.

Pain can be quite an attention getter! Pain can be reinforced and rewarded by health-care professionals who greet it with attention and medication. Pain medication taken on a regular schedule is more beneficial than taking it on an as-necessary basis (PRN) because you want to avoid rewarding the pain by taking medication on a PRN basis. Likewise, you are better off resting when you still feel all right, rather than waiting for fatigue to knock you down.

It is healthier to listen to the wisdom of your pain signals than to make them your main focus, ignore them or totally numb them out with medication. Make them your guide and not your god.

Learning from Your Pain

All kinds of pain – physical, mental, spiritual – are trying to tell or teach you something about yourself. Your pain is telling you that you need to change something. Ask yourself questions about the pain. Are you focusing on physical pain to avoid your family's emotional or spiritual pain? Is your physical pain hampering your ability to cope with emotional challenges? Learn from the pain, and change your life.

PART IV

Making Changes

CHAPTER 20

Mind/Body Maintenance

Everything in this life is subject to wear and tear. Watches, computers, appliances, houses – almost all offer warranty contracts to cover the possibility of malfunction or break-down. Your car's good working condition depends on routine maintenance checks.

Adequate rest, a well-balanced diet and exercise are all forms of maintenance for your body. Physical checkups, including a pap smear or prostate exam, and dentist's visits, among other tests, are probably included on your calendar at regular intervals.

You rarely think of maintenance for your emotional health. It's a medical fact that stress affects your emotions and your body. You can't treat one without treating the other.

Stress is experienced both emotionally and physically. The two responses cannot be separated. A change of temperature, a loud noise, success or failure, pain or pleasure, boredom or overstimulation – almost anything can produce stress, resulting in a change in the chemical balance of the body, among other reactions.

When you are stressed, your body prepares to either stand your ground and fight, or turn and run in flight. This physical readiness includes dilated pupils; increased heart rate; faster and deeper breathing; increased blood pressure; tense and contracted muscles resulting in an accumulation of pyruvic and lactic acid (waste products from muscle activity); blanched skin; and excretion of norepinephrine (an adrenal hormone) into the system.

Chronic stress can produce other more distressing effects such as headaches; gastrointestinal problems; back and neck pain; chronic fatigue; high blood pressure; restlessness, irritability and frustration; decreased zest for life; worry, fear and depression; decreased performance and efficiency; difficulty making decisions and forgetfulness; increased use of alcohol, cigarettes or drugs; eating and sleeping problems; disease flares; and poor immune system function.

Hans Selye, the father of the study of stress, has written that we all have a limited amount of energy to adapt to stressful situations. When your adaptation energy is gone, you're at risk of breaking down physically, emotionally or both. People with chronic illness start out higher on the stress scale than people who aren't ill, and so may be more susceptible. It takes less to stress you and you'll feel the stress more than you did before illness.

Too much stress can translate into illness as the body continuously tries to adapt. Stress of a biologic or emotional nature is known to exacerbate and prolong disease activity in many chronic illnesses – some of which may have been initially triggered by stress.

Stress can be caused by pleasant as well as unpleasant events, although stress caused by unpleasantness usually lasts longer and causes more problems. Stress is an unavoidable and integral part of life. If managed properly, it can be a friend; if ignored, a fatal enemy.

If your perceived resources are equal to your perceived demands, you are confident and active. You're smoking! If your perceived resources are not equal to your perceived demands, you're under stress – distress. You need to eliminate demands, increase resources or do both to regain balance. Listen to and learn about yourself from your stress.

Thirty years ago, researchers thought major life events (divorce, death, job change, marriage, promotion, pregnancy) had the most effect on your likelihood of becoming ill. The more major life events you encounter, the more likely the impact on your health would be negative.

Major life events (such as the diagnosis of a chronic illness) results in everyday hassles (taking medications, going to the doctor, dealing with medical insurance). These hassles have a great effect on your health. Major life stressors may have such a large impact because they translate into a multitude of continuing hassles.

The effects of stress tend to accumulate over time, resulting in a stress spiral. When you are stressed, an event that you ordinarily might not respond to sends your stress level even higher. With the next stress, you start out at a higher level, going even higher. Your chances of recovery from the stress spiral diminish with each succeeding stressor. Failure to recover may lead to both physical and emotional problems.

With the population in general, stress can become such a

way of life that its effects are no longer recognized. You may even become addicted to stress. Unaware that you've steeped yourself in tension, you may not even know what it is like to really relax.

With chronic illness, your body is constantly stressed. Emotional and social stresses also multiply. Smaller irritations may matter more.

More than the average person, you need an ongoing means of stress recovery. Building stress maintenance and release into your life every day is critical for your health.

Stress management needs to be individually tailored to each person's requirements because everyone reacts differently to stress. What stresses me may not stress you. What relaxes you may not relax me. One formula won't work for everyone or all situations. Stress management can work in a number of ways, either through prevention, by handling the aftermath, by becoming stress hardy, or by all three approaches.

Richard Lazarus at University of California, Berkeley suggests you can actually balance out the effects of stress if you have two "uplifts" (uplifting experiences, ranging from a pleasant time with your family to getting enough sleep) for every hassle you go through. You may have to consciously plan to incorporate such sources of enjoyment into your life. Studies have actually shown fewer disease flares with a better hassle:uplift ratio (one hassle to two uplifts).

HASSLES SCALE

Hassles are irritations that can range from minor annoyances to fairly major pressures. Listed here are a number of ways in which a person can feel hassled. Go through the list and put a check by those hassles that have happened to you in the last month. Then, add up you total score. Ranking your perception of your hassles and uplifts on a scale of 1–3 can give you more information. Compare to the score on your Uplifts Scale. Aim for getting an Uplifts score that is at least twice your total Hassles score.

1. Misplacing things
2. Trouble with neighbors
3. Social obligations
4. Health problems of family member
5. Concerns about debts
6. Smoking too much
7. Drinking too much
8. Trouble relaxing
9. Trouble making decisions
10. Problems with people at work
11. Customers or clients give you hard time
12. Home maintenance
13. Concerns about job security
14. Don't like current job
15. Bored
16. Lonely
17. Fear of confrontation
18. Illness
19. Unhappy with physical appearance
20. Sexual problems
21. Wasting time
22. Problems at work
23. Car trouble

24. Rising prices
25. Not getting enough sleep
26. Problems with your children
27. Problems with your parents
28. Problems with your spouse or lover
29. Too much to do
30. Work unchallenging
31. Legal problems
32. Concerns about weight
33. Not enough energy
34. Feeling conflict over what to do
35. Not enough time for family
36. Property, investments or taxes
37. Yard work
38. Concern about news
39. Crime
40. Traffic
41. Pollution

Other hassles, not mentioned yet:
42.
43.
44.

Modified with permission of Richard Lazarus.

UPLIFTS SCALE

Uplifts are events that make you feel good. They are sources of your contentment, satisfaction and joy. Put a check by any events that may have made you feel good in the last month. Then add up your total score. Compare to the score on your Hassles Scale. Aim for getting an Uplifts score that is at least twice your total Hassles score. Once again, ranking your perception of the uplift on a 1–3 scale may give you more information.

1. Getting enough sleep
2. Being lucky
3. Saving money
4. Not working
5. Having pleasant conversations
6. Feeling healthy
7. Being with children
8. Visiting, phoning or writing someone
9. Relating well with your spouse or lover
10. Completing a task
11. Being efficient; meeting responsibilities
12. Cutting down on smoking
13. Cutting down on drinking
14. Losing weight
15. Good sex
16. Friendly neighbors
17. Eating out
18. Having plenty of energy
19. Relaxing
20. Having the "right" amount of things to do
21. Good times with friends
22. Spending time with family

23. Buying things for yourself or your house
24. Home pleasing you
25. Giving or getting a present
26. Traveling
27. Doing yard work
28. Making a friend
29. Getting unexpected money
30. Dreaming
31. Pets
32. Children's accomplishments
33. Things going well at work
34. Making decisions
35. Confronting someone
36. Being alone
37. Knowing your job is secure
38. Feeling safe in your neighborhood
39. Fixing something
40. Meeting a challenge
41. Flirting

Other uplifts, not mentioned yet:
42.
43.
44.

Modified with permission of Richard Lazarus.

Emotions play a part in how you react to stress. Most people aren't taught how to express anger or deal with depression or anxiety. You may have been unconsciously taught to bottle up negative or messy feelings so you didn't rock the family boat!

Becoming aware of and modifying your perceptions, expectations, or beliefs can turn a potentially stressful event, accompanied by hammering heart and sweaty palms, into a neutral event producing little or no stress.

How you choose to combat stress may depend on how you respond to it. People generally respond to stress either mentally or physically, or by some combination of the two. Sometimes the first step to learning how to successfully handle stress is listening to your body, so that you can better understand how to reduce the effects stress is having on it.

In the mental response, the person becomes fixated on the problem, ruminating on it continually. Physical response is exhibited by muscle tenseness, sweating and increased blood pressure, pulse and respiration.

For those who respond to stress mentally, techniques are aimed at breaking the compulsive thought pattern – taking your mind off the stress. For those who respond physically, the recovery strategy uses physical change to break or release body tension.

The next few chapters of this book will examine techniques for handling stress.

Remember that gentle is the way. It's taken you a lifetime to get where you are. It takes 30 days to break an old habit and put a new one in its place. It'll take time, patience and perseverance to discover and reinvent yourself and ways of handling your sources of and reactions to stress.

1. List things that stress you.
2. How do you handle stress now?
3. What demands or hassles can you eliminate?
4. What resources or uplifts can you add in?

CHAPTER 21

New Year's Resolutions

Promises, the saying goes, are made to be broken. Did you ever make any New Year's resolutions? Did you write down these promises to yourself? Did you calculate their cost in time or effort, or plan how you might go about implementing them? Or did they just quickly cross your mind?

One worthwhile resolution for the chronically ill person is to learn more about your sources of stress, how stress affects you, how you can avoid it, and how to handle it. As defined in the last chapter, stress results from anything that forces you to use energy to adapt to it, emotionally or physically. Once your adaptation energy is exhausted your health may suffer, so it's especially important for the chronically ill to work on reducing stress.

Some techniques aim at teaching you to calm your response to stress. Methods such as meditation, relaxation and biofeedback work to replace your quick response to stressors – sort of like replacing a gun's hair trigger with a harder-to-squeeze model.

These calming techniques reduce your level of arousal, and give you a quiet sense of control. Eventually your entire attitude may be affected. You may still experience stress, but less readily, and you will recover from it more quickly.

Other techniques are more physical, aimed at burning off stress, along with the wastes and toxins it may produce (such as pyruvic acid, lactic acid and norepinephrine). Psychosocial stressors that you encounter daily in being a family member, an employee or employer, or just a human being, usually involve no physical activity to flush the effects of stress out of your body. It might take days for the toxins and muscle tension caused by a brief argument to be absorbed and flushed from your body without some physical action.

A side benefit of these physical methods, such as noncompetitive exercise (working out to tapes or as your doctor directs you, walking, swimming, stretching, yoga), is a deep sense of relaxation, as well as increased body awareness and hardiness. Your emotional reactivity is reduced and the intensity of your stress response is minimized.

Stress Recovery Approaches

If you respond to stress more physically than mentally, some recovery approaches for you might include aerobics, bicycling, dancing, deep breathing, isometric exercises, jogging, massage, sex, swimming, walking, hot tubbing or golf. Each of these approaches involves either working tension out of muscles or relaxing them.

If you respond to stress more in a mental manner and less physically, you might try counseling, cultural events, getting together with friends, keeping a journal, music, crossword puzzles, reading, support group, computer games, putting puzzles together, television, meditation or surfing the net. Each of these activities involves either distraction, quieting the chatter of the mind or processing what's going on in your head.

Those who respond to stress both physically and mentally might try autohypnosis, biofeedback, martial arts, meditation, primal screaming, sex, video games, yoga or yelling while beating up on a pillow.

Invoking the Spirit

Dealing with chronic illness needs to be a mind/body/spirit effort. Leaving out the spirit, that part of you that makes you feel alive, omits an essential ingredient. (The mind/body/spirit connection is explored fully in Chapter 32.) Turning to spiritual forms of relief is valuable for many in handling stress.

Follow your own spiritual path, but such methods could include prayer, reading inspirational material, singing hymns, sharing your life and story with other people, counseling, meditating, worshiping and drinking in the beauty and wonder of nature.

Resolving to Change

Your main New Year's resolution needs to be putting your health first on your list. That means doing all you can to reduce your stressors and take care of your stress responses. For each person that may be different and change with each day's level of disease activity. Any gain is worth the effort.

You're in charge: Decide you'll make some of these suggestions your New Year's resolutions. You don't need to wait until New Year's Eve – just remember that the day you begin will be the start of a whole new year for you.

CHAPTER 22

Lifestyle Engineering

In the next two chapters, we'll look at ways to make changes in your life to reduce stress. Lifestyle engineering adjusts the way you live – your schedule, work, diet, social life, recreation. Personality engineering adjusts your attitudes and thought processes.

Taking Responsibility

"I'm sorry, but I can't give you any more medication," the doctor wisely and thoughtfully utters. "Although what you are experiencing is frustrating and painful, at this point it isn't life-threatening and doesn't warrant the side effects that more or different medication or treatment would include. To some degree, you'll just need to learn to live with it. Change your lifestyle, and see if that helps."

Those wise and thoughtful words may be hard for you to accept and even harder to implement. You adopted a lifestyle early in your life that matched your personality (see the next chapter) and helped you get along in your family and feel safe and useful. The five most prevalent lifestyles according to lifestyle theorists are the pleaser, who lives to please others; the perfectionist, whose self-worth is based on success and competence; the victim, who feels he has no control over his life; the controller, who fears the worst and constantly prepares for it; and the martyr, for whom each molehill is a mountain.

Yes, it is hard to change a lifestyle you adopted as a child. Hard, but not impossible. After you become ill, assuming responsibility for yourself means sometimes you'll need to intentionally change the ways you've always done things. Lifestyle engineering can help.

Your lifestyle generally focuses on three major tasks of life: building social relationships, intimate relationships and career. Each of these areas is full of stressors: giving parties, writing reports, disciplining the kids, shopping. Then there are environmental stressors such as diet, heat, cold and noise. Changing your lifestyle can alleviate some of the effects of these stressors.

The primary goal in lifestyle engineering is not to change the stressors, but instead, to modify your association with the stressors. For example, if you find it particularly stressful to work with a particular person, you have three options: to limit the amount of time you spend with him, to change your physical proximity to him by moving your desk, or to remove yourself completely from all involvement with him.

Lifestyle engineering can be as simple as getting out of bed earlier or driving to work by a different route or as difficult as finding a new career, mate or life goal. You may have the misconception that you have to live a stress-filled life, when in reality you actively seek out a stressful lifestyle because it offers more money or prestige. You may even be addicted to stress because it gives you a certain high.

Don't mistake addressing the sources of your stress and changing your relationship to them as running away. It's not stoic or macho to work outside in the blazing heat if you know it aggravates your illness. You may have to work first to recognize your stressors, because of a sense of invulnerability or denial.

Some people avoid stress by withdrawing from life. Others do nothing to change their stressors. The ideal balance is somewhere between these two extremes. Maintain a healthy respect for stress and manage it with the path of least resistance.

Some stressors are irritating to almost everyone; other pet peeves are uniquely your own. Find out what pushes your buttons.

Possible Sources of Stress

Frustration

Frustration explains most common, everyday stress. Frustration arises when a desired goal or behavior is inhibited – you can't do or accomplish what you want. To understand the source of your frustration, understand why the goal or behavior is desirable to you. Be as specific as possible.

For example, if you're frustrated because you feel unfulfilled, decide what concrete things, people or events will make you feel fulfilled. Use realistic goals. If your illness has forced you to stop some activities, such as working full-time, that gave you a sense of accomplishment, you may now have to focus on another method of achievement. It may take education, counseling, time and patience to unearth this information about yourself.

Overload and Boredom

Deadlines, extra responsibility, lack of support and overly optimistic expectations all play a role in overload.

One way of relieving overload is managing time better. Prioritizing, problem-solving, pacing and planning can help a great deal. I practice the four P's all the time.

Using the four P's, I can accomplish my goals – travel, write, maintain a heavy schedule – while suffering the least consequences to my health. Research has shown that the chronically ill perform best when they have the flexibility to control their schedule, work environment and demands.

Another method of relieving overload is learning to say no. Delegating responsibility or asking for help may be difficult because it may mean giving up prestige and power. The benefits to your health will be worth it.

You may find that you give up less prestige than you'd anticipated by wisely sharing a workload. Knowing your limits, what stresses you most and why, enlisting others' help and accepting your own (and others') fallibility will go a long way toward preventing overload. You are free only when you know your limits. Otherwise, you are chained to the consequences of your unrealistic goals.

Boredom can be just as stressful as overload. Lack of stimulation, activity and connection with life can cause your health to spiral down. The chronically ill may find boredom to be a particularly thorny enemy because your active life may have been curtailed against your will.

Plan some relaxing activities that aren't competitive or mentally complex to fill up the time when you may need to slow down. If you were like a racehorse charging through your old life, you may need help in adapting to your new one.

When I have down time or a molasses day, I enjoy working jigsaw puzzles, doing crewel or handwork, reading, talking to friends on the phone, writing letters, watching TV, renting movies and catalog shopping. Find and keep on hand what you need for your own special hobbies or activities that spark life for you. Pick them up anytime you hit the wall and need to fill the activity gap.

Schedule Changes

Changes or novelty, even when connected with happy events, produces stress because they take up more adaptation energy. Such stress can be avoided or modified by synchronizing your biologic rhythms with your schedules and routines. Biologic rhythms, such as sleep cycles and times of peak energy, may wax and wane more erratically with the chronically ill. These changes may require you to listen to the new illness-related messages your body is sending you and adjust your schedules to their wisdom.

You may have been a morning person in the past but now find it impossible to get up and going at the crack of dawn. Don't force yourself: Listen to your body and find out when it's most comfortable to get up. You may need 12 hours of sleep now instead of eight. You may now have to plan around being functional two or three hours a day instead of eight to ten.

Synchronize your social clock with your biologic clock. If you feel most relaxed and ready to talk in late afternoons, plan your phone conversations with friends then. Routines and behavior patterns provide a framework by which you can balance your life and reduce stress. As your routines become automatic, you use less psychic and physical energy.

Reserve specific time periods for certain tasks on a daily or weekly basis. I run errands on one day a week, and limit them to maybe four in the same area of town. I write in my prayer journal and listen to inspirational music in the morning as I try to get going and at night as I try to wind down.

Set aside one day of the week as a "mental health day." Don't schedule anything you don't enjoy that day, and make it as simple and relaxing as possible. A full day of reading, light exercise, napping, eating and laughing may go against your workaholic nature, but it actually may be good for you.

Because of the changes in your schedules and rhythms, vacations may actually produce stress for you. They also mean you have to find your bearings in a new environment, which also takes energy. Don't rely on a vacation to reduce your stress and relax you.

When your life is already full of turmoil and change, avoid making changes other than those you absolutely have to. Examine the many individual stressors in your life, and choose your battles wisely.

Biologic and Environmental Stresses

Just living in this modern age can be stressful: You may be surrounded by noise, allergens, pollution, bright lights and junk food. But you can fight or avoid many of these unhealthy influences.

Begin with your diet. If you live alone or work too much, it's easy to take in too much caffeine, eat fast foods or too much sugar and salt, and develop a random schedule of starving and then stuffing yourself. All are unhealthy.

Seek out a well-rounded diet, and supplement with vitamins and minerals, if necessary. Refined flour and sugar add stress to your body because they are harder to digest than whole grains and unprocessed sugars. Reducing salt, caffeine and artificial sweetener intake is also healthier. See your doctor if you need help establishing a diet plan.

To reduce allergens and pollutants in my house, I have found that HEPA filters on my heat and air systems are effective. I carry a portable water and air filter with me when I travel. I even wear a small air purifier around my neck that puts out a clean airflow to my face. It has helped a lot.

Noise, too, can produce physical and psychological stress. Research shows that too much noise can produce cardiovascular changes, tissue damage in the inner ear, an increase in stress hormones, reduced concentration and lowered patience. Try ear plugs, or if your bedroom is noisy try a "white noise" machine (or turn on a fan, vaporizer, TV or radio at a low volume). Many cars now advertise their quiet interiors as a selling point. Once you start looking, you'll find other ways to quiet your life.

Balancing Resources and Demands

Stress can throw you off balance. You can work on your stress with lifestyle engineering by learning about your resources and demands. Balance is the goal.

Some resources you can use to reduce stress include finding social support, becoming physically fit, having a realistic attitude toward your financial circumstances and becoming assertive, among others.

With any chronic illness, medication can help only so much. In fact medication can add adaptive stress, or other toxic effects on your body. Lifestyle engineering helps to create the balance between demands and resources that you need to get better.

Medication only allows the body to do its own work.

I've lived with lupus for 20 years. I still have my ups and downs but I am doing the best I've done, and on the least amount of medication! I believe it is because I've learned what works best for my mind, body and spirit and I use that program daily. Medication, I think, is only about 10 percent of the answer. Learning to make lifestyle and personality changes are the other 90 percent.

I've gone from "musterbating" to needs, wants, likes, thinks, feels; living from the inside out instead of the outside in.

It may take a long time for you to learn how to balance your resources and demands with lifestyle engineering to handle your stress effectively, but you can do it. You gain control of your destiny by learning about the boundaries of your freedom. Remember: It's up to you.

CHAPTER 23

Personality Engineering

Personality engineering deals with the way you look at things, the meaning that you attach to events, and your expectations of life, self, others and your Higher Power. An event may be neutral or stress-producing, depending on how you interpret it. You can't and don't want to change your personality. You can fine tune and become as healthy as possible in your personality.

Your personality is a composite of your values, attitudes and behavior patterns, determined long ago by your heredity and environment. Your personality determines your lifestyle: If you're the kind of person who approaches life aggressively, you're more likely to have a busy, high-stress lifestyle.

Stress expert Hans Selye has said that by adopting a healthy attitude toward life, you can turn harmful distress into positive stress. Personality engineering can help.

How Do You Look at the World?

As discussed in the last chapter, a lot of stress is caused by frustration – being unable to do something the way you want to. You can either change your lifestyle – your relationship to what frustrates you – or you can change the way you look at it.

Being diagnosed with a chronic illness is stressful, and at times of stress, your personality traits and behaviors may become unhealthy and your lifestyle more fixed and rigid. It may be time to evaluate the way you look at the world.

Philosophers and psychologists have come up with many different ways of describing personality types. The Enneagram is a modern synthesis of ancient ways of looking at personality. Nine personality types are grouped by three main Triads, centered around the heart, head and gut, otherwise known as Feeling, Thinking and Instinctive Triads. Types within the Feeling Triad include the Reformer, Helper and Motivator; types within the Thinking Triad include the Individualist, Investigator and Loyalist; types within the Instinctive Triad include the Enthusiast, the Challenger and the Peacemaker. If you want to learn more about Enneagrams, you might try one of the following books:

Baron, Renee and Elizabeth Wagele. *The Enneagram Made Easy: Discover the 9 Types of People.* New York: HarperCollins, 1994.

Baron, Renee and Elizabeth Wagele. *Are You My Type, Am I Yours?* San Francisco: HarperCollins, 1995.

Riso, Don Richard and Russ Hudson. *Personality Types: Using the Enneagram for Self-Discovery.* New York: Houghton Mifflin, 1996.

Riso, Don Richard and Russ Hudson. *The Wisdom of the Enneagram: The Complete Guide to Psychological and Spiritual Growth for the Nine Personality Types.* New York: Bantam Doubleday, 1999.

THE ENNEAGRAM

The Enneagram has been a helpful tool for me to discover my personality type. It gives me a map and a mirror that describes behavior and traits that let me know when I'm descending into unhealthy levels of my personality ... a helper or Number 2.

The Nine Personality Types of the Enneagram

1. THE REFORMER: The principled, idealistic type.

2. THE HELPER: The caring, interpersonal type.

3. THE ACHIEVER: The adaptable, success-oriented type.

4. THE INDIVIDUALIST: The introspective, romantic type.

5. THE INVESTIGATOR: The perceptive, cerebral type.

6. THE LOYALIST: The committed, security-oriented type.

7. THE ENTHUSIAST: The busy, productive type.

8. THE CHALLENGER: The powerful, aggressive type.

9. THE PEACEMAKER: The easygoing, self-effacing type.

Key Terms for the Helper

HEALTHY: Level 1 – Self-nurturing, unconditionally loving

Level 2 – Empathetic caring

Level 3 – Supportive giving

AVERAGE: Level 4 – Well-intentioned, people-planning

Level 5 – Possessive, intrusive

Level 6 – Self-important, overbearing

UNHEALTHY: Level 7 – Self-justifying, manipulative

Level 8 – Entitled, coercive

Level 9 – Feel victimized, burdensome

Reprinted with permission by Don Riso and Russ Hudson of The Enneagram Institute, 212/932-3306

Researcher Albert Ellis, a pioneer in rational emotive therapy, and others theorize that psychological problems can be traced to illogical thinking. The following eleven erroneous ideas or beliefs can create stress in all of us. These are the beliefs that Ellis identified in many emotionally and psychologically disturbed people.

1. I must be loved and appreciated by everyone in my community, especially those who are most important to me.
2. I must be perfectly competent, adequate and successul before I can see myself as worthwhile.
3. I have no control over my happiness – it is completely controlled by external circumstances.
4. My past experiences have determined my present life and behavior – the influence of the past cannot be changed.
5. There is one right and perfect solution to each of my problems. If it is not found, it will be devastating for me.
6. Dangerous or fearful things are causes for great concern and I must be prepared for the worst by constantly dwelling and agonizing over them.
7. I should be dependent on others and have people stronger than myself on whom I can rely.
8. If life does not work out the way I had planned, it will really be terrible. When things go badly for me, it is a catastrophe.
9. It is easier to avoid certain difficulties and responsibilities than to face them.
10. Some people are bad, wicked and villainous and should be blamed and punished.
11. I should be very upset over the problems and disturbances of other people.

Anxiety seems to develop predominantly from the first seven ideas and hostility from the final four.

Ellis divides these major beliefs or ideas into three "whines," in which something is "awfulized":

1. Poor me! ("Awfulizes" oneself)
2. Poor, dumb other people! ("Awfulizes" what others are doing to me)
3. Poor, dumb life and universe! ("Awfulizes" what the world is doing to my life).

To read more about Ellis' theories, read *Fully Human, Fully Alive: A New Life Through a New Vision* by John Powell (Thomas Moore Press, 1989).

When you're ill or alone, your thoughts can be stressful. Check the list below to see if you recognize any of your "tapes" in these unhealthy patterns (adapted from David Burns: *Feeling Good: The New Mood Therapy*. Signet, 1980). The following thoughts can lead more to depression or be an expression of being depressed.

1. All-or-nothing thinking: You view the world in black or white, good or bad – extremes with no middle ground. You think of yourself as all good or all bad, and not a mixture of both. One experience, negative or positive, may unrealistically color your total outlook on life or yourself.
2. Overgeneralizing: One single negative event may be seen as a never-ending pattern of defeat.
3. Mental "filtering:" You pick out one negative part about yourself or your life and dwell on it exclusively, and it darkens the rest of your vision of reality. When you are depressed you block out anything positive.

4. Disqualifying the positive: When you are depressed and something positive happens, you ignore or dismiss it as not being significant. You aren't able to embrace or absorb a compliment, good news, an award, success, victory or achievement. You dismiss it as a fluke or maintain that it doesn't count.

5. Jumping to conclusions.
Mind reading: You assume you know how people are feeling and what they are thinking about you. You may then react by withdrawing or counterattacking when the person's actions may have nothing to do with you.
Fortune telling: You imagine negative or bad things as about to happen and foretell only misery for yourself. You take this as a fact and act on it even though it may not be based on reality: A friend doesn't return a call, so you feel angry rather than checking to see if she got the message. One negative lab test spells doom.

6. Magnifying (catastrophizing) or minimizing: You either blow things out of proportion or shrink them, depending on which end of the binoculars you are looking through. You magnify your errors, fears, limitations and imperfections and exaggerate their importance.
You may magnify other people's positive or good points. You minimize and play down anything good or positive about yourself. Inferior feelings are guaranteed to follow.

7. Emotional reasoning: You use your negative feelings as the only test of reality: "If I feel this way, it must be this way." Your conclusions, based on your negative reasoning, aren't based on reality.

8. "Musterbating": You punish yourself or others with "should,

ought, must, got-to/have-to" statements instead of using "need, like, think, want, to feel" statements. If you or others don't perform under this pressure, resentment, shame, blame and guilt result.

9. Labeling: As an extreme form of overgeneralization, you may in anger apply a label to yourself or someone else. The label is usually a judgment response to the self or other's behavior that colors your reactions to yourself or others. I'm a "pig," he's "insensitive" or "uncooperative."

10. Personalizing: You assign yourself great powers to control, not just influence, others. You assume responsibility for negative events even when there is no reason for doing so. You blame the responses of other people on your sense of inadequacy rather than allowing them to be responsible for their own actions. You feel crippling guilt and carry the weight of the world on your shoulders.

Everyone thinks these unhealthy thoughts from time to time. If you find yourself living these tapes, you need to find a balance.

Finding a Balance

Don't assume that you have to be a Pollyanna to be happy. Healthy thinking includes positive and negative thoughts ... or maybe two positive thoughts for each negative.

If you want to try to find the distortions in your world view, you're going to need to be willing to face facts, whatever they may be. It is not easy to accept your own shortcomings. You'll also need to admit to a credibility gap between who you really are, who you pretend to be or who you would like to be. Act on your insights to make them permanent.

Victor Frankl, the concentration camp survivor and psychiatrist referred to earlier, suggests that another essential ingredient in discovering your vision is letting life question you. For instance, the needy person who threatens to exhaust your patience silently asks, "What limits do you put on your love for me?" An enjoyable experience asks, "How capable are you of enjoying life?" A suffering loved one asks, "Do you believe you can grow and go through hard times?" Your response to these questions gives a candid picture of your vision.

What questions is your illness asking you? What lessons do you have to learn about yourself from your illness? If you don't learn these lessons, they'll come back again and again, exacting a greater price each time.

Personality Engineering Techniques

Your personality determines how you handle events, thereby producing or reducing stress. Some psychologists feel that the basis for personality is firmly fixed by the age of 5. However, other psychologists suggest that you can change your beliefs or attitude about yourself and your experiences.

The major personality-related causes of stress are self-perception, "Type A" behavior and anxious reactivity. Being honest with yourself about your attitudes and beliefs will enable you to go beyond them. You can then address each of these personality-related causes of stress with specific strategies.

How Do You Look at Yourself?

The way you feel about yourself – your self-esteem – is one of the greatest factors influencing your behavior. Research shows that the devalued, helpless and hopeless self-concept (a totally passive and dependent role) produces increased stress that can lead to illness.

Responding to stress with a feeling of helplessness, hypervigilance, and withdrawal is called passive coping. This unhealthy attitude can affect you physically, resulting in mental depression and immune system suppression.

Active coping – assuming responsibility for yourself and acting on your own behalf – can actually change your body chemistry for the better. You can modulate your mood and pain levels by the way you to respond to stress.

Accepting yourself as a blend of strengths and weaknesses, and embracing all aspects of yourself (without labeling them as good or bad), is a healing experience. This experience is not short-term and one-time, but an ongoing renewal. A lifelong process, self-acceptance adds greater enrichment as time goes on.

Positive self-concept can be the difference in whether a person survives or succumbs to an illness. Underrating yourself and just focusing on the negative aspects of your life can result in a poor self-concept. Balance out the negative with positive verbalization and affirmations, acceptance of compliments and assertiveness.

Realistic, positive verbalization and affirmations reinforce your self-concept by pointing out the positive. Affirmations, which are used widely in 12-step programs, are short quotes or maxims that help you keep perspective, such as the Sanskrit proverb, "Look to this day, for it is life," or the Scottish saying, "Better bend than break." You can find books of affirmations in most bookstores, and of course you can find thoughts that have special meaning for you in whatever you read for inspiration, such as the Bible.

Verbalize the positive by saying good things out loud. Or write yourself positive messages: "You lost five pounds! Congratulations!" "You balanced the checkbook! Hurrah!" Put them on a calendar or on note cards in a conspicuous place where you can see them and be proud of yourself.

When others give you a compliment, accept it without adding minimizing statements, such as "Oh, thanks, but it's nothing, really." Instead, add statements of agreement – "Thank you! I enjoyed doing it!" – to improve self-esteem.

Assertiveness – somewhere between passivity and aggression – lays the groundwork for you to appreciate yourself and to think more positively about yourself.

Assertiveness can be practiced in daily contacts. Greeting others, giving compliments, using "I" statements to own how you feel ("I need help with some errands today," as opposed to "you" statements, such as, "You never help with the errands"), asking "why," spontaneously expressing feelings, disagreeing with someone you feel is wrong, and maintaining eye contact are all ways to assert yourself.

One way to practice assertive responses is to frame them into three parts. The first part is the empathy statement. You state what you understand about the other person's situation or feelings, using, "I understand that you ..." Second, state what you need, want, like or think. Finally, ask for what you need, set your boundary or negotiate your solution.

For example: "I understand that you want to go to a movie and then dinner, but I feel really hungry, so I'd like to go to dinner first." Or: "I understand that you don't feel well, but I feel it's important for me to go to this meeting, so why don't you rest and I'll come back to get you later." You may need to repeat your assertive statement over and over like a broken record. You need to be clear, specific, direct, kind and firm.

From Type A to Zzzzzz

Maybe you know a "Type A" individual: This person is aggressive and sometimes hostile; always seems to be under a deadline; is intensely ambitious; and often tries to accomplish many tasks at once. Maybe you *are* a Type A.

Type A behavior isn't a temporary response to a stressful situation. It's a well-ingrained behavioral style that constantly triggers the stress response that leads to cardiovascular arousal. Heart and other physical problems may be seen more often in this person.

Type A's can alleviate their stresses from deadlines with better time management. Research has shown that Type A's, for all their motion, often accomplish less than those who aren't as driven because they try to do too many things at once, resulting in time-consuming errors. Prioritizing and allocating blocks of time for tasks, making lists, or assigning things for specific days can help, as can rewarding yourself when tasks are finished.

Type A's can calm themselves by developing the ability to concentrate on one thing at a time. Focusing purely on the mechanics of a task, and not constantly analyzing performance, helps alleviate stress and avoid errors.

If you're a Type A, try to make yourself complete a task before going to another one. Realistically evaluate your time urgency, and go back in this chapter and check the thoughts that may drive you. It may be helpful to realize that your work is separate from you. It is acceptable not to have all the answers, and it is only human to have limits or to be ill.

Fighting Anxious Reactions

The anxious reactive person experiences stress long after the event that triggered it – sometimes the stress even grows with time. This kind of reaction can cause psychosomatic disorders, or even mental and physical incapacitation, from the slightest stress.

Your thoughts can create a volatile mind/body feedback loop. Reliving or "catastrophizing" an event over and over after it has happened generates ever-greater anxiety and ever-greater bodily responses. Your body doesn't know the difference between the actual event and your thoughts about the event. It reacts the same way to both.

Keeping a diary can help you become aware of what your thoughts are and if they are healthy or unhealthy. Once you identify the unhealthy thoughts, you can catch yourself and use a "thought-stopping" technique.

Thought-stopping is an attempt to break the vicious cycle of obsessive thoughts. One method is saying, either to yourself or out loud, "Stop!," as soon as you become aware that you are reliving or catastrophizing. Another method is to wear a rubber band around your wrist and snap it when you become aware of your reliving or catastrophizing. Why don't you try one of these thought-stopping techniques tomorrow? Get out a rubber band (not too tight) and give it a chance for a day or two.

Another way to break the cycle is to train yourself to immediately switch your focus to a pleasant scene once obsessive thinking begins. Use the same scene each time, focusing on it for 30 to 60 seconds. Repeat the visualization until the cycle is broken. This can be a powerful tool, but it does take practice.

Deciding to "Redecide"

Learning about your personal style and making unhealthy, unconscious behavior conscious so you can change it, is all a part of becoming as healthy as you possibly can. A moment of "redecision" can free you to make those choices. Becoming as healthy as possible in your personality can take a long time, but it can be both successful and rewarding. Replacing stressful behaviors with consistent, constructive, less stressful patterns will lead to a healthier, happier life, despite the presence of chronic illness. This process will take patience, willingness to experience pain, humility, courage, silence and solitude, a questioning spirit, determination, experimentation and practice.

You can discover new possibilities only by breaking down old barriers. It's your choice. Only you can decide to redecide!

CHAPTER 24

Replacing the Hair Trigger

Have you ever felt that if you had to deal with one more problem, your head might just snap off your neck and go spinning off into space? Or if someone said one word the wrong way to you, you might just enjoy jumping down his throat? If so, you are a normal person who's been under a lot of stress.

Everyone experiences a stress spiral, where each successive stressor sends you a little higher on the stress scale. The more stressed you become, the harder you find it to relax.

Chronic illness adds stresses while lowering your abilities to cope with them. It takes less to cause you stress and you feel the stress more than the average person.

Just as a gun's hair trigger must have its spring loosened to help reduce its sensitivity, you can reduce stress intensity with relaxation techniques. Meditation, biofeedback, deep muscle relaxation and breathing exercises are a few techniques that can increase your stress threshold.

Meditation

Many religions advocate some form of meditation, which has been practiced for more than 7,000 years. The key element of all meditation techniques is shutting down thoughts, since thoughts produce emotional and physiological arousal.

Your body can't rest until your mind is shut off. Your mind is working even when you are asleep. Meditation is similar to staring into space, with your mind thrown out of gear. Have you ever arrived home and realized you can't remember driving the last stretch of the trip? Meditation is a bit like that, except the state is attained intentionally and maintained for a prescribed period of time.

You learn to focus on a stimulus that has little arousal for you, allowing feverish thinking to slow down, and producing a calmer, more centered consciousness. The focus is different from person to person and from time to time in the same individual, because of changes in what produces arousal. Life's noise is quieted, and you become aware of your spirit and body in the present moment.

According to measures taken during meditation, the body's basic metabolic rate slows 16% to 17%, carbon dioxide elimination increases, the respiratory rate decreases, oxygen is used more efficiently, and blood lactate levels that produce anxiety are decreased. Heart rate and blood pressure both drop. These physical changes aren't just limited to time you spend meditating but carry over to other times of the day.

Psychological responses are also affected. Meditators respond to stress just like anyone else, but recover from stress better and don't get caught in the stress spiral as often.

In Eastern thought, meditation broadens perception, decreasing the emphasis on ego. Egocentricity is often a source of stress.

People who meditate say they achieve a greater sense of self-love, patience and a sense of peace. In India, the mind is often compared to a drunken monkey that produces useless, erratic thoughts and internal noise that shut out awareness. Research has shown that any major stress – such as chronic illness – can result in jumbled thinking. Meditation's purpose is to quiet life's chatter, get you past your ego, and open you up to a new awareness of yourself and the universe.

Harvard cardiologist Dr. Herbert Benson has developed a relaxation exercise that he feels produces the same effects as meditation. The exercise involves concentrating on breathing patterns while saying the word "one" to yourself upon exhalation. Benson contends that the exercise's full effect won't be felt until it is used for a month, one to two times a day for ten to twenty minutes. See Benson's relaxation technique in Appendix A.

Deep Muscle Relaxation

Every time you think of carrying out a motion, the muscles that you would use tense up. Muscle tension is left behind. For instance, if you are thinking of saying a word, your vocal chords move just like you are saying the word. Stress is stored in your muscles as tension. That tension causes you to exert even more tension to carry out a task.

Excess muscle tension can be an expression, as well as a cause, of stress. You may not even be aware of your muscle tension because it is so subtle and difficult to detect.

Anxiety and tension from everyday stress, coupled with the stresses of chronic illness, can bring on a chronic state of muscle tension. Muscle tension has been linked with disease and pain for hundreds of years. But only since the end of the last century have relaxation programs been formulated.

Muscle tension by itself can contribute to and worsen your physical condition, including pain and fatigue. It can also drain your precious energy reserves and keep you from falling asleep or sleeping deeply.

There are many different types of muscular relaxation techniques, all of which teach you how to relax muscles at will. To do this, you first need to be taught to feel the difference between being tense and relaxed. Some people may be wound so tightly that they need to exercise and do deep muscular relaxation before they can attempt any meditation techniques.

Try to practice muscle relaxation twice a day – morning and evening are best for most people. Practicing in the morning often helps begin the day less feverishly. Practicing in the evening helps you wash out the cumulative stress of the day and go to sleep.

Try one or both of the two similar muscle relaxation techniques that are in Appendix A.

Breathing Exercises

When you're stressed, your natural breathing rhythm is interrupted. Hyperventilation or hypoventilation may result. Hyperventilation is rapid, shallow breathing, resulting in increased oxygen intake and decreased carbon dioxide levels in the blood. Dizziness, weakness, the numbness of an extremity, nervousness and many other frightening physical responses may result. The responses of your body and mind create even more anxiety.

Hypoventilation is marked by slow breathing, resulting in decreased oxygen intake and increased carbon dioxide levels in the blood.

The philosophy of yoga contends that the mind is master of the senses, while the breath is master of the mind. Breathing exercises can strengthen and condition your pulmonary system, enhance your cardiovascular system, promote oxygenation and calm your nerves.

The reticular activating system (RAS) is the part of your brain that filters any stimuli reaching the brain. It is your security system, which decides if a stimulus goes any further in the brain. The brain's breathing center is very close to the RAS. Constant, steady, restful breathing will also calm the RAS and promote relaxation.

Your stress spiral can be broken by using any or all of these techniques. Each technique may not be appropriate for every person, but you won't know if anything works for you unless you try it. You may find that you need to scrape yourself off the ceiling less often.

A meditation technique that includes deep breathing and muscle relaxation can provide a greater sense of relaxation and restfulness than taking a nap. A nap can actually leave you feeling more tired and drained and throw off your sleep for the night.

Deep breathing, relaxation and meditation played a big part in my finding a sense of peace, calm and focus while living with chronic illness. These techniques have opened me up to emotional and spiritual growth I didn't know was possible.

CHAPTER 25

Me? Exercise?

Exercise?! I have a chronic illness! I get tired just walking to the mailbox! I'd rather save my energy for other things! Perhaps you've heard these responses to the suggestion to exercise – perhaps they've come out of your own mouth.

Let's take a look at some of the effects of activity and inactivity.

According to NASA, bed rest can cause a dramatic decline in the physical condition of perfectly healthy people. Lying in bed for long periods of time actually adds to the aging process. After you've been in bed 18 hours, your heart gets smaller and blood volume is reduced. After three days, you lose muscle tone, get flabby and start to waste away. Your bones lose calcium and you start dehydrating.

After prolonged bed rest, you'll feel faint upon getting up, because of a drop in blood pressure. With each day you spend horizontal, the condition worsens. Staying in bed is tempting when you feel bad, but you'll shorten your convalescence by trying to get up as soon as possible. The unhealthy effects of being flat on your back are reversible. There are exercises you can even do in bed.

Fatigue can actually breed fatigue. If you resign yourself to inactivity (which slows down the functioning of your autonomic nervous system), you'll only end up feeling more tired.

Research shows exercise (and exercise alone) provides a wide array of benefits, including better joint flexibility; stronger muscles and ligaments; stronger bones; better cardiovascular conditioning and circulation; better balance and coordination; release of antihistamines to relieve inflammation in joints; improved stamina; bowel regularity; better sleep; release of endorphins, providing pain relief and a natural high; faster metabolism for easier weight loss; reduced fatigue; improved mind/body connection ... and more!

Usually, fitness and health go together, but it is possible to have a serious health problem and be physically fit in terms of muscle tone, flexibility and maybe cardiovascular endurance. Being fit also allows you to be more stress hardy – an important physical and emotional benefit for the chronically ill.

Studies show a correlation between regular exercise and improvement in depression, anxiety, hostility, social interaction and outlook for the future. Exercise can play an important role in improving your self-image, as well as giving you a sense of accomplishment and control. Your fears about the strengths and weaknesses of your body will also lessen as you gain a sense of mastery over your physical abilities.

Working out helps you work off stress, along with the toxins it produces. It's actually more stressful to watch an athletic event than to participate in it! The athletes are burning off the anxiety you feel as your favorite team tries desperately for that last-minute winning goal.

Developing an Exercise Program

There are three parts to a balanced exercise program: warm-up, endurance and cool-down.

Warm-up includes range-of-motion, stretching and strengthening exercises. Warm-up exercises safely prepare your heart and lungs for endurance, nourish your joints and help maintain or increase flexibility and muscle strength.

Endurance exercises, also called aerobic exercises, use the large muscles of the body and are important for cardiovascular fitness, weight control and for lessening fatigue.

Cool-down exercises help the body relax and let you lose some of the heat you generated while exercising. Cool-down includes aerobic exercise done slowly, followed by flexibility and stretching exercises.

Flexibility and Range-of-Motion Exercises

These exercises reduce muscle stiffness and help keep your joints flexible. Move your joints through their full range of motion every day, even when you are taking a break from your aerobic routine. A sustained, gentle stretch to tight muscles will assist in relaxing that muscle, thereby improving flexibility and reducing pain.

Strengthening Exercises

Strong muscles help keep your joints stable and more comfortable. Two common types of strengthening exercises are isometric and isotonic. In isometric exercises you tighten your muscles but don't move your joints. An example is when you tighten the muscles in your buttocks, and release, and tighten, and release. In isotonic exercises you move your joints against gravity or against some mechanical resistance. An example is doing leg raises or lifting dumbbells.

Endurance (Aerobic) Exercises

Endurance exercises strengthen your heart and make your lungs more efficient. They lessen fatigue by giving you more stamina, helping you sleep better, controling your weight and lifting your spirits. Walking at a rate that allows you to continue talking is an example of aerobic exercise.

If you exercise beyond your level of fitness, you'll end up with sore muscles, pain and fatigue. If you cannot talk while you're exercising, you may be working out beyond your physical limitations. Slow down a bit but don't quit.

With chronic illness, your level of fitness may change from day to day and hour to hour. One day, your level of fitness may allow you to make it to the bathroom and back. Another day, you may be able to walk up and down the mall.

GET FIT

Frequency (how often): New guidelines for good health recommend some kind of moderate physical activity on most days of the week.

Intensity (how hard): Exert yourself at low to moderate intensity. At maximum you should be only slightly out of breath. If you can't carry on a conversation, count out loud or sing because you are working too hard, you are overdoing it.

Time (how long): Guidelines recommend about 30 minutes of aerobic activity on most days. You may have to start with several sessions per day of only a couple minutes each. Gradually build to three 10-minute sessions and then to 30 minutes all at once. This may take months.

Cautions

The activity you choose needs to be individually tailored to your situation, level of physical fitness and interests. Your limitations may wax and wane with your condition – you may need bed rest in times of increased disease activity, and at other times you may be able to engage in vigorous aerobic exercise. All you may be able to do is range-of-motion or toning exercises. Do what you can.

Keep in mind the Zen aphorism, "Gentle is the way." You may need weeks, months or years to build up your strength, and it could be some time before you notice a reduction of stress. Don't expect too much, too soon.

Activity can be, in itself, a stressor. The exercise needs to be noncompetitive, even with yourself. A competitive mind is stressful. Don't compare what you can and can't do now with what you used to be able to do or what someone else can do. Try to refrain from self-evaluation. What you are trying to do is kindle a fire that will increase circulation and burn off stress byproducts.

You may wish to focus on exercises that work around problems your illness may present – such as sore joints. Low-impact exercises such as walking, stretching and yoga may work best for you. Try them. Be creative.

Listen to the signals of your body.

Any activity on a regular basis is better than none. Some days, that may be anything from wiggling your toes in bed to water aerobics – whatever suits you best at the time.

Exercise needs to be something you enjoy or you won't follow through with it. Working exercise into your daily schedule or activities can be helpful. Park your car at the far end of the parking lot or take the stairs when you feel up to it.

Ask your doctor about some form of exercise and what limits you need to observe. Weigh the advantages and disadvantages of each kind of exercise. Above all, listen to your body and the messages it sends you. It may take a lot of time and patience. Even at that, things will fluctuate.

Find Your Pace

There's a risk involved with everything in life – even in trying to exercise. But the greater risk may be remaining inactive and sedentary. You may add to your illness and aging process by not exercising.

If the exercise you try makes you feel worse, you may have tried to do too much. Don't give up. Try something different and do less. When disease activity flares, you may lose ground. Keep trying.

My doctors can testify to what it has and is still taking to find the best activity for me day by day. It takes determination and endurance to keep on keeping on. My efforts are paying off. I've been tempted to give up at times, but I haven't. Neither should you. Good luck!!

CHAPTER 26

Holiday Blues

Holidays are a potent stew of traditions, scrambled schedules, increased activity, altered demands and heightened emotion. People with chronic illnesses, already moving more slowly than the general masses, may find themselves even more outdistanced by the quickened pace. Carefully arranged schedules, made to conserve energy, are often tossed aside.

These special days may bring on extreme highs and lows, great happiness and deep depression. Blessings and losses are magnified. It can be a sober time for reflection. You might take some time to think about where your life is and what is really important.

You may become acutely aware of your losses – health, goals, ambitions, functions, loved ones or changed relationships. You may feel that others are blessed by so many things that your life seems to lack. You may even have lost touch with some of the ways you expressed your love to those important people in your life.

At the same time, you may need to travel to family gatherings, see more people than usual, prepare larger meals – just generally do more and be more excited about doing it. Any way you look at it, your time, energy and ability to cope may be challenged.

Why consider all this? Well, maybe you have experienced the holiday blues. This might be a good time to sit back and evaluate what contributed to them. From there, you can decide how your holidays can be handled in a healthier way that accommodates your limits but also expresses your uniqueness.

Finding New Traditions

Through the years, you may have established ways of expressing yourself during holidays by the gifts you give, the foods you cook, the time spent with family and friends, and community or church activities you attend. These traditions, etched in time, have become a part of your life.

As chronic illness invades your life, you may need to handle those traditions differently. Normally, age changes holiday customs, as family dynamics accommodate transitions and the passage of time. Chronic illness may bring about these changes more swiftly.

It may be difficult to give up customs that have become extensions of yourself. At Christmas, I found that singing the carols I loved caused excruciating pain from the chest inflammation that often accompanies lupus flares. Decorating the house would stir up dust, increasing the chance of life-threatening infections. Trying to cook big meals for large family gatherings drained all my energy.

So I re-evaluated my Christmas celebration: I learned I could sit down and sing one verse at a time without triggering pain. Instead of trying to put up a tree the way I'd done in the past, I trimmed my whole house as if it were a tree, putting decorations on every doorknob, light or edifice. I limited the size of gatherings at my house, and made easy "tursghetti" (spaghetti with ground turkey, sausage and beef) to allow guests to feed themselves. And as for Christmas cards ... sometimes I send Easter cards instead. I have more energy and money in the spring!

It's important to remember what holidays are all about. Your children or siblings may have to take on certain customs, such as cooking or decorating or serving or shopping. Or perhaps the customs themselves will change. You may decide you like Chinese takeout and a video as your New Year's Eve celebration. Perhaps you will, with great fanfare, hand over your matzo recipe to your daughter-in-law (or your son the chef!) in time for Chanukah. Keep the meaning and spiritual value of these important days, but don't be afraid to change the way you spend them.

Making Other Changes

Physical and emotional expenditures exact a price from your well-being. When holidays demand more physical and emotional energy than you have resources for, you'll have to decide if you can afford the cost.

Holidays are a time to enact some of the lifestyle and personality-engineering techniques mentioned in Chapters 22 and 23. The four P's (planning, pacing, problem solving and prioritizing) may also help you minimize your efforts and maximize your enjoyment. Here are just a few specific suggestions:

1. Shop by catalog. Mail-order houses can do it all, including wrapping and mailing directly to the recipient. You can now find catalogs for just about anything, including food.

2. Simplify meals. Let each guest bring a dish. Whole meals can be catered, if necessary. Precooked turkeys and hams can be purchased with side dishes included. You may also be able to freeze some of your favorite dishes, which would allow you to prepare them far in advance of the crush.

If possible, plan family gatherings at someone else's home. When this isn't possible, don't hesitate to delegate some responsibility to others. When you do, remember that everything doesn't have to be done the way you've always done it!

Let your helpers make the kind of stuffing they like, set the table the way they want to, and do the cleanup according to their system. So what if you can't celebrate the way you once did? Being together is the important thing, even if you gather around paper plates. Recognize your limits, and don't be embarrassed to seek out a quiet place to rest during the hubbub.

3. Don't spend the holidays completely alone. Find someone to spend a little time with, even if just on the phone. Whenever possible, capture the magic of the season. Find your own unique way to reach out to others, staying within your limits. Be good to yourself on special days and find ways to celebrate holidays as well as every day of the year.

4. Let whatever time you are together be special. I try to create a holiday spirit for myself rather than expecting it to come to me from other people. I let my grown children know my days will be simple, fun and happy.

I want to see them when it works for them and have them join my holiday spirit. I don't want to send them on a guilt trip if they can't be with me on that special day. Any day we get together is special.

My oldest son, Jamie, comes to town at the first of January. We celebrate my December and his January birthday, Christmas and the New Year all together. I make sure to give myself good gifts physically, emotionally and spiritually. I'm only good for other people when I'm good for myself and can give myself good gifts.

5. Tell people what you want or need. During holidays people may run away from you, forget you or try to rescue you by coming up with an endless list of things for you to do that they think may cheer you up but really just anger and exhaust you.

They may be well meaning, but they try to force things on you without asking what you want or need. You may already be short on energy without extra activities. Some may try to "save" you, to insist you spend holidays with them so you won't be by yourself. If you want solitude, and prefer to keep in touch with others via phone on those days, say so.

Figure out for yourself what makes a holiday special for you and let others know, whether it's music, candles, lights, a hot dog, fireworks or parades. I saw three sets of fireworks on TV this last Fourth of July, from Boston, Baltimore and Washington. I was glued to the set for every minute of it and joined along singing at the top of my lungs with every patriotic song that I knew the words to. My puppy was horrified!

6. Take care of your pain and fatigue. Take pain medication and rest on a regular schedule before and after increased activity. If your pain and fatigue become severe, you'll need to work even harder to recover. I go into exercise training to get ready for trips and holidays so I'll be more stress hardy.

7. If your holidays were difficult last year, try not to repeat the same mistakes this year. Insanity is the same damn thing over and over. Sanity is one damn thing after another! Try to keep moving ahead.

   If you feel emotionally stuck or stagnant, you may feel even more so during holidays. As a result, emotions you've being trying to repress, suppress or deny may come exploding to the surface. You also may be trying to cling to old traditions that don't work now, resulting in more anguish.

Letting Go and Moving On

So much of life is letting go. Breathing, laughing, crying, giving birth, singing ... all require letting go. Grieving your losses, celebrating victories, growing emotionally – all these also require letting go and going with life's flow. You hurt yourself by holding on.

To enjoy the holidays now, you may need to let go of the way you spent them in your old life. Keep some of the old, but create new traditions and ways of being a family. You may find this way of living healthier than your old "healthy" life.

I have found that chronic illness has served to sharpen my experience of the holidays. I've needed to slow down, recognize, appreciate, treasure, enjoy and celebrate precious relationships and all of my blessings. I've learned the joy-dance of life.

CHAPTER 27

Music Therapy

Throughout the ages, music has been a balm to the wounded spirit and a salve to the ailing body. In the Old Testament, King Saul had the shepherd boy, David, play his harp to soothe him.

Modern-day medicine now uses music as a therapeutic tool. Neurobiologists recently discovered direct evidence that music stimulates the parts of the brain responsible for memory, motor control and language. Those researchers now believe music may be able to "retool" brains with some neurological disorders.

Dentists who supply their patients with portable radios and headphones have long known that music can provide a distraction, reducing anxiety and stimulating the release of endorphins, the body's own painkillers. Some people have formed "music therapy groups" to meet and sing together – performance isn't important – for the solace it gives.

Music is powerful! The music people listen to has been

blamed for crimes they committed. Gov. Zell Miller of Georgia pioneered a program to issue classical-music CDs to parents of the state's newborns, because research has shown that listening to Bach and Mozart enhances babies' intellectual development.

Music vibrates the chords of your soul as nothing else can, expressing the full symphony of emotions – reverence, anguish, joy, defeat, anger. A song can cross cultural, language and age barriers to speak to whole crowds of wildly diverse individuals. When one of our Olympic athletes climbs on the pedestal to receive a gold medal, American spectators of all ages and races swell with pride as they hear the national anthem. Grown men cry.

Music has always had a significant place in my life. I always sang in choirs. As a teenager, at night I would go out on the roof of our home. I'd sing – old favorites and songs I'd made up – to the stars, moon, clouds, animals. I was embarrassed to learn later that my neighbors would come out and sit in their back-yards to listen!

Today, after I speak, I sing a song that seems to sum up the theme. It often seems to reach people in the audience who appeared unaffected by my presentation up to that time.

Music has perhaps played an even greater role in my life since chronic illness announced itself. I try to fill my every moment with some kind of music. The amount of disease activity, to some degree, determines the beat I can tolerate.

Exercising to music is a lot more fun – and goes faster – than without it. You may also find you'll gain a sense of agility and coordination that carries over even after you've finished.

When I hear a peppy song, I dance around the house like Fred Astaire or Ginger Rogers for a two- to three-minute range-of-motion workout, much to my puppy's bewilderment. I keep my radios throughout the house and in my car tuned to stations that play upbeat music.

Music can stimulate and comfort you no matter where you are. During one hospitalization, I enjoyed playing my John Denver tape and harmonizing with it – while in bed, in the tub or the hall! It was my high spot on days when I was feeling pretty low.

My radio and tape player are musts when I pack for the hospital or travel, ride in the car, get ready for the day or go to bed.

My tastes run to Celine Dionne, Gloria Estefan and Whitney Houston. Songs like "I Made It Through the Rain," by Barry Manilow and "Sweet, Sweet Surrender," "Today" and "Rocky Mountain High," by John Denver are my pick-me-ups. "Climb Every Mountain," "The Impossible Dream," "Be Thou My Vision" and "Amazing Grace" put to music thoughts and themes that have become important in my life. They became songs of my heart throughout my struggle with chronic illness.

Of course, you may be rolling your eyes at these choices – pretty much the way my sons did when I turned up the volume to my music on the car radio. Maybe you're not a singer, or a musician of any kind. But you can still reap the benefits of listening to, and fully enjoying, your favorite kind of music.

If you never had time to really explore the world of music, or if you've never really thought about who you like to listen to, now's your chance! You have an exciting world of musical discoveries ahead of you.

Finding the kind of music that blows *your* horn is half the fun. Once you do, fill your days with it – opera, rap, folk, polka, big band, classical, Aretha Franklin or Frank Sinatra – there's a wide realm of music out there waiting to comfort and challenge you in a way nothing else can. As you listen, you'll feel less pain, and more alive.

What will be the soundtrack to your life's "movie"?

CHAPTER 28

Me? See a Shrink?

Somewhere along the line, someone may suggest you see a counselor. Whether a doctor, a family member or a friend makes the suggestion, you may perceive it as criticism. You may think it means you're somehow weak and unable to cope. You may be convinced you don't need that kind of help.

For many, going to a psychiatrist or psychologist is taboo. It's an option never to be discussed, much less exercised. My mother's emotional difficulties were a carefully guarded secret even after her death. Some family members resisted having her courageous battle with manic-depressive swings mentioned in her funeral eulogy. They'd only allow a general reference to Mother's heroic lifelong struggle.

The counselor is an important member of the medical team that treats the chronically ill patient. It is difficult to admit the need to see a psychiatrist. Somehow, it's easier to deal with doctors who specialize in physical problems – a nephrologist for kidney ailments, a dermatologist for a rash – than to see a doctor or counselor who is trained to work with emotional issues.

Your emotions not only control how you feel and interpret things, but also affect the level of your disease activity. When you get stuck in heightened emotions, such as anger, anxiety or depression, they may turn on, stir up and prolong disease activity, and can affect its severity.

The expense of getting counseling may be a heavily weighed factor in deciding whether to pursue the referral. Medical expenses may already be sapping your budget. But I feel adjustment to a chronic illness is 10% physical and 90% mental. A trip to a counselor may actually save on medical bills in the long run. Some insurance covers psychiatric visits, with certain limits. Check with your provider.

Physical complaints can overshadow the emotional problems that may have triggered them. Anxiety and depression can cause rapid heartbeat, poor appetite, fatigue, hyperventilation, increased urinary frequency, insomnia, skin rashes, muscle tension, shortness of breath, diarrhea, constipation, headache, indigestion, hypertension, and many other problems.

It is sometimes difficult for a physician to determine how a physical problem relates to an emotional problem. Psychiatry is the branch of medicine that is concerned with the body's function as a whole, both physically and emotionally. The physical, mental and spiritual are intimately interwoven, each affecting the others. You may see a psychiatrist so he or she can determine how your physical and emotional states are interacting. You may then get referred on to a psychologist, counselor, marriage and family therapist, social worker or chaplain for one-on-one therapy.

When I was having a flare that involved respiratory problems, my physician suggested that I see a psychiatrist. My first
reaction was one of hurt and anger. I felt I had been coping
pretty well with all the turmoil that chronic illness had
dumped into my lap.

The suggestion came across to me as, "I don't feel you're
handling this very well – maybe you need some help." It made
me feel that he didn't think my respiratory complaints were
based on real, physical problems, but were only a manifesta-
tion of my anxiety.

I let some time elapse before the actual referral was made. I
went back to some of my nursing textbooks and reviewed the
overlapping effects the emotions can have on the physical self.

Slowly, I began to realize how difficult it is to weed out the
intertwined effects of emotions on your physiologic functioning. I could see the strain the many adjustments to chronic illness were putting on me, my marriage and my family life.

As chronic illness and different medications exert their
effects, personality changes can occur. Your personality as it
was before becomes magnified, both the good and the bad.
You'll be the same as you were before illness, only more so!

If a psychiatrist had never met you and didn't know you
prior to changes due to illness or medication, how could he
know what behavior was new and what was old?

I realized seeing a psychiatrist might be a chance to grow in
self-understanding and I wanted him to get to know me
before the effects of illness and medication had changed me
too much. I decided to see that shrink – maybe it was a good
idea, after all.

On my first visit, there was no couch to lie on, as I had

anticipated, only comfortable loveseats to sit on. The atmosphere was very relaxed. For two one-hour sessions, I had the opportunity to open up and share all of the hurts, adjustments, fears, anxieties, worries, hopes and dreams I was experiencing and their relationships to my illness, in a nonstop stream of communication that helped me to put together thoughts that had been fragmented.

The psychiatrist understood the devastating effect that losing control has on the ego, the strain of changes made in lifestyle, the fear of the unknown related to illness, and the disrupting effect a sudden hospitalization has on an individual and family. Almost every aspect of my life was and would continue changing in some ways.

Very carefully, he picked out small crystals of thought and held them up for me to examine. Looking at them closely, I could see where, in some instances, I was exerting my energy and getting nowhere. He helped me to understand my situation and to cope with it a little better.

I discovered some things about myself. I realized that I do worry a lot, and admitted it to myself. Before, I had always justified it under the guise of being a mother, or being a nurse, or being in charge. By admitting to myself that I do worry, I was also able to acknowledge that worrying never changes anything but me. It's a futile, self-defeating activity.

I decided to write down everything I worried about. I even worried about worrying! The uselessness of it all dawned on me and helped me to shed some of it.

Other aspects of my life became clearer. I recognized the importance of keeping communication lines open, with my counselor and with others; that I'm not responsible for other people's reactions or responses to me, nor can I change them; that I need to be myself. I learned that talking through problems helps bring them into better perspective and shrinks them down to size; that some anxiety and depression is normal, but I can find my way out of them; that emotions affect illness; and that whether from a psychiatrist or other counselors, therapy can help.

If I get into deep water emotionally in the future, whether from my illness, reaction to drugs, or family or social problems, I feel that my psychiatrist or counselor knows me and I know him. I wouldn't be going to a stranger. He could better determine what was going on with me.

I left my shrink's office with the understanding that I would return if I experienced depression that I couldn't bounce back from, if thoughts of my illness and its effects became a preoccupation, or if family problems became difficult. It was up to me.

We finally determined that my breathing problems were a result of many things – exertional asthma, sinus congestion, inflammation of the lung and heart linings, deconditioning and emotions. I constantly work to take care of all of these sources.

In going through my divorce, my two sons and I entered family counseling. Those sessions made it possible for us to get through an impossible time. We even learned something about ourselves and grew. Today, I'm amazed at some of the healthy things my sons say and do.

I hope that I have learned some healthier patterns of behavior and relating that will help them be healthier in their lives and relationships. What a wonderful gift counseling for illness and divorce may have given me! I'm still in recovery from codependency, but maybe I can pass that gift on to future generations.

CHAPTER 29

A Journey Inward

My world was neatly arranged – everything was in order, with schedules to live by and plans for the future. I felt that I really had it all together. Hard work was paying off in success and personal fulfillment as a wife, mother and career woman.

My life was full. I felt I could perform all my family, work, church, community and school commitments with one hand tied behind my back. I was, after all, the Enjoli woman – just like the beautiful model in the commercial who could do it all and still be sexy at the end of the day. I even wore the perfume.

From out of the blue, chronic illness struck and my whole life was transformed right before my eyes. Chaos replaced order – schedules were made only to be broken, and plans for the future were replaced by a mist of vague uncertainty.

Sometimes a whole day would be spent just struggling to get up, get dressed and then stay up. The Enjoli woman, able to handle it all, was transformed into the Geritol woman, with tired blood.

Days that were once filled with activity were emptied. I just existed, moving from bed to couch to hospital and back again. Although my body had been halted, my mind raced. Thoughts bumped into one another, chased about by fear, uncertainty, anger, guilt, grief and confusion.

Without all those plans and schedules to give structure to my days, I really wasn't sure who I was anymore. What were once priorities – helping other people, entertaining, constantly staying on the go, climbing the ladder of success – no longer were possible for me.

One of the ways I made sense of my racing thoughts was to write about them in a journal.

Writing It Down

As a young girl and teenager, I had been a faithful diary keeper, filling a couple of five-year diaries with reminiscences of my growing-up years. It's fun today to read those young impressions and remember the experiences and stages of growth.

Little did I know that I was developing a practice that would help me salvage my sanity in later years. Keeping a journal helps me make it through the storm of chronic illness back into the sunshine, and even find a rainbow along the way.

After I became ill, I instinctively returned to and expanded that journal-keeping habit of my childhood. I began writing down my thoughts, emotions and feelings evoked by turbulent events in my changed life. I thought of my entries as letters to God. I often call my journal a "prayer journal." Whether you consider your journal a conversation with a higher power, or your inner self, writing your thoughts helps clarify them.

My thought patterns were often fragmented, and at times, obsessive. Writing them down forced me to put them into some kind of order, and allowed me to carry them through to completion. At times, it was the only way I could work my way through a problem or sort out the answer to a question.

Sometimes I'd find deeply moving insights into some of my most distressing emotional struggles. But even when I didn't find answers, simply expressing a thought, worry or fear in its entirety often released it. I was freed to turn to other tasks.

My journal has become much more than just a record of my days. It has become an inner journey to find and accept myself, warts and all. Like many journeys, this sojourn isn't about arriving at a destination, but about what happens along the way: the process. It helps give me perspective and find deeper meaning in my life.

I may have lost certain physical abilities, and may be poor as the world judges wealth, but through keeping a journal, I am becoming rich in self-awareness. In doing so, I tap into my own inner wellsprings of joy, peace and celebration.

Letting It Out

Repressed or unacknowledged feelings can be lethal to the soul. Whether feelings are unconsciously blocked, or repressed out of fear, guilt, pity or some misguided urge to protect the self or others, it really makes no difference.

Those suppressed thoughts and feelings will find expression somehow, and they may well emerge as physical symptoms or destructive behavior. You can actually make yourself sick by denying and holding onto your feelings. Even if you don't become ill, at best you cease to fully live and experience yourself.

Getting in touch with your feelings can be scary. Sometimes they may feel so strong you fear they will sweep you away. I've found, however, that if I allow my feelings and their accompanying truths to wash over and toss me about, I feel cleansed afterwards.

Benefits of Keeping a Journal

Studies have shown you can exhaust an emotion by going into it, embracing it and moving on. Research has also shown that people who write down their thoughts and feelings or talk about them into a tape recorder see improved health: Immune systems are strengthened by better T-cell functioning.

Keeping a journal puts you in touch with your feelings – sometimes even those you don't want to acknowledge. You peel them away layer by layer. Facing them in the privacy of your diary allows you to acknowledge flaws you want to correct in yourself. Perhaps you would never have realized that your animosity toward another family member was based on jealousy if you hadn't examined your writings.

Your journal can become a sort of "paper psychiatrist," helping you sort out emotional problems. The best effect of your writings is catharsis – you find an outlet for your emotions and get in touch with your own wisdom. (For more help on making personality changes, see "Personality Engineering," Chapter 23.)

Writing in a journal allows you to harness your thoughts and emotions and use them constructively rather than letting them run away with you.

Keeping a journal is a form of meditation. Don't content yourself with merely thinking about what you might write – it's not the same thing as writing it. Writing evokes depth that thinking does not reach.

Thinking about problems rarely allows you to organize your thoughts about the problem's facets and ramifications. Just as talking with someone else will suddenly allow you to focus more clearly, keeping a journal is like holding a conversation with yourself. It can serve the same purpose of clarification.

Getting Started

First, find the method of writing that feels most comfortable to you. Do you like typing, writing longhand or talking into a tape recorder? Once you decide on a method, you will want to make it as comfortable as possible. Choose your favorite materials – like a yellow legal pad and black roller-ball pen, or favorite word-processing program – and settle in. Find a cozy place and some privacy. Turn the TV off. I always play some music and light candles.

You may find that keeping a journal works best when you write at the same time every day. Whether that's first thing in the morning or the last thing at night, it really doesn't matter. Allow yourself at least 15 minutes to jot down your thoughts.

If you find it hard to get started, try focusing on something small that happened that day, or a problem that's been on your mind recently. You don't need to try to solve the problem, or to paint a huge landscape – just try for a small snapshot. Details are sometimes more important than obvious facts.

Again, if you have trouble, just work on keeping your pen moving – don't let your inner "editor" tell you what's not worthy of jotting down. Write down your activities, events, problems and spontaneous emotional reactions.

You may find that you like keeping a journal so much that you will write longer than 15 minutes. I try to make it easy to write wherever and whenever the mood strikes. In addition to the 500-page ledger journal I keep by my bed, I carry small journals in my car, purse and tote bag so that anytime I am waiting, I can pick up my pen. I sometimes splurge on special, fancy journals for traveling.

However you decide to record your thoughts, the important point is to jot them down on a regular basis. Remember, when your mind is spinning, it's dragging your body around after it. Stop now and write what you are thinking and feeling at this moment.

Checking It Out

Over time, you may or may not want to go over what you wrote and assess it honestly. As you check out and challenge the validity and reality of your beliefs and thoughts, you'll see if your emotional reactions are in healthy proportion to the event, problem or circumstance.

The more precise and vivid your written descriptions are, the greater the chance that misconceptions, unhealthy thinking and unrealistic expectations will surface to be recognized.

Suspend your inner critic and absorb what you've learned about yourself in the mirror of your journal and apply it to your life. In this way, you may gain new insights and challenge unhealthy ingrained emotional patterns. Your perceptions may broaden as you grow and your emotional reactions change.

Resources

Ira Progaff, a psychologist, stumbled into the benefits of

keeping a journal during an emotional crisis in his life. In the upheaval following the separation from his wife and the loss of his two children, he began writing in a notebook.

He found he was able to get a fix on his life by writing things down. He used his journal to keep a "dialogue" with himself, his wife and his children.

Progaff came up with a formal way of keeping a journal that he began teaching in books and workshops. These workshops are available throughout the country today. If you are interested in learning about keeping a journal, this would be an excellent place to start.

Progaff's *At a Journal Workshop* (JP Tarcher, 1992) is a great book to begin with. You can learn more about Progaff's work and workshops by contacting 1-800-221-5844, 1-212-673-5880, or www.intensivejournal.org. My experience with the Progaff method has been most beneficial for me in refining my understanding and practice of keeping a journal.

Other books that might be helpful are *The Vein of Gold,* by Julia Cameron (Putnam, 1996) and *The Long, Quiet Highway,* by Natalie Goldberg (Putnam, 1994).

A Clean Slate

My journal helps me untangle the web of my confused thoughts and emotions. Writing them down frees me from my useless obsessional ramblings to redefine the dimensions of my vision of reality. Keeping a journal helped me make the transition from Enjoli woman, to Geritol woman, to who I am today – the Enjotol woman, still capable and valuable, but who knows her weaknesses as well as her strengths, a human being not a human doing.

When I'm writing, order replaces my chaos, my fears are

quieted, uncertainty is cleared up, my anger is defused, my guilt is recognized, and my confusion is replaced by clear thinking. I can leave my struggles there on that stark piece of white paper and go in peace.

Journaling has become my bridge to emotional and spiritual freedom. I integrate insights and understandings and give birth to new beginnings. I don't really leave anything behind or change my circumstances. My inner world, that is inescapable and goes wherever I go, is drastically and beautifully altered and stretched.

CHAPTER 30
Reading Therapy

When I was a kid growing up on a farm, I probably would have responded to a suggestion to read with, "Me, read a book?! You've got to be joking! I'd rather be out riding my horse, swimming or playing ball with the guys. Books are boring!" I was too busy trying to be Annie Oakley to read!

Even when I grew up, I didn't care much about reading. While at Vanderbilt University Nursing School, I read only the required material. I was too busy doing things and dating the man I was going to marry to spend a lot of time reading.

There was even less time to read after we married and our two sons were born. I worked to put Jim through eight years of school for his master's and doctorate at the seminary. I was also carrying out the many functions of pastor's wife and mother.

When chronic illness invaded my life, I suddenly had a lot of time on my hands. Without much energy to do anything, I knew only that I had entered a whole new way of living that I knew nothing about. I needed to learn how to exist with this new reality in as healthy a way as possible. I began reading everything I could get my hands on, but there wasn't much available.

From my reading, I realized that along with my physical illness, I had also adopted an unhealthy "sick role." Depressed, frightened and anxious, I was allowing my emotions to worsen my symptoms.

Reading turned out to be one of my footholds on stability, as everything in my life seemed to shift and change. Books not only filled my time, they filled my mind with words of wisdom, comfort and inspiration, as I heard the echoes of my own experience captured in the writings of others.

Setting my own pace, I began to discern and understand truths about my changed reality and aspects of myself that I had never needed to face before. I became acquainted with a blend of the old and new me.

Here are some quotes from books that helped me along the way.

To Kiss the Joy (1977, Word Books)

This book, written by Robert Raines, was one of the first I read after I became ill, through the fog of a clouded, confused and troubled mind. It touched my wounded spirit and continues to bring me joy each time I read it. In it I found what has become my goal for living: "To kiss the joy of life as it flies is to live in the Spirit, it is to live boldly, immediately, with gracious abandon, daring to risk much, willing to give one's self."

To me, this joy, life, was symbolized by a fleeting, delicate butterfly. If I held on to it too tightly, it would be crushed. If I opened my fingers and released it, I would be rewarded with the awesome sight of its flight.

Another of my favorite quotes from this book: "To go with the flow of your life is to live without a map ... to be vulnerable to having your mind and plans changed, your heart broken, your dreams fulfilled. It is to trust that God is in the rapids of change as well as the rocks of continuity. It is being able to stop digging your heels in against the tide of tomorrow."

Although this book is now out of print, it was important enough to me in my journey that I wanted to mention it anyway. You may still be able to find it in your local library or through special order at a bookstore.

On Borrowed Time (Medical Economics Co.)

Dr. Samuel Chyatte's book describes his own journey with diabetes and end-stage renal failure. It touched me profoundly. In it, I learned, "Denial isn't all bad. I'm sick, but I keep going. I push away all the implications of my illness so I can function today. That's useful denial. Depression and tears seem to be the mechanism that restore the grieving to normalcy."

His insights into relationships of the chronically ill provided me with a much-needed bridge of understanding. He summed it up by saying, "Keep a humorous perspective on your illness that tells your plight and leaves them smiling."

With the honesty of one who has been there, he touches on the topics of children, family, doctors, marriage, sex and work, as they become entangled in the web of chronic illness.

Although this book is now out of print, it was important enough to me in my journey that I wanted to mention it anyway. You may still be able to find it in your local library or through special order at a bookstore.

Man's Search for Ultimate Meaning (1997, Insight Books)

Jewish psychiatrist Victor Frankl describes his own experiences as a survivor of a Nazi concentration camp. It includes these thoughts:

"The attempt to develop a sense of humor and seeing things in a humorous light is some kind of trick learned while mastering the art of living."

"A man who lets himself decline because he could not see any future found himself occupied with retrospective thoughts. In robbing the present of its reality lay a certain danger. It becomes easy to overlook the opportunities to make some positives of camp life, opportunities that really did exist."

"It is a peculiarity of man that he can live only by looking to the future ... sudden loss of hope and courage can have a deadly effect. ... Human life under any circumstances never ceases to have meaning, and this infinite meaning includes suffering and dying, privation and death."

Getting Well Again (1992, Bantam)

Carl and Stephanie Simonton and James Creighton have written from their experience about the effect the psyche has on illness, especially cancer.

"We all participate in our own health through our beliefs, our feelings, our attitudes toward life, as well as more direct ways, such as through exercise and diet. The individual who assumes the victim stance participates by assigning meaning to life's events that proves that there is no hope."

"By recognizing your own participation in the onset of your illness, you acknowledge your power to participate in regaining your health and you have also taken the first step toward getting well."

"It is our central premise that illness is not purely a physical problem, but rather a problem of the whole person, that includes not only the body, but mind and emotions. Expectancy, either positive or negative, can play a significant role in determining an outcome."

The Healing Journey (1992, Bantam)

Carl Simonton, MD, went on to write this book with a patient, Reid Henson, who survived a type of cancer usually considered incurable. Henson's story of healing is interlaced with medical and scientific data along with emotional issues.

"I believe that the power of the mind goes far beyond what I first imagined. In addition, I believe that, beyond the mind and body, there is another aspect of healing that needs to be addressed: the spiritual aspect."

"The dictionary defines spirit as the life principal, especially in humans, and the feeling and motivating part of our lives. The mind alone can be used to influence the physical state, it is used most effectively when it is aware of the spirit."

"An idea that I found enormously helpful in making healthy changes was to assume the perspective of 'student of life.' As a student of life I became an independent observer of myself. I began to practice seeing each event in my life as a learning opportunity. Life is the teacher. I am the student."

Although this book is now out of print, it was important enough to me in my journey that I wanted to mention it anyway. You may still be able to find it in your local library or through special order at a bookstore.

Healing Words: The Power of Prayer and the Preactice of Medicine (1993, Harper)

Larry Dossey, MD, wrote this book to help restore the spiritual art of healing to the science of medicine.

"The impulse to *do* when sick is understandable ... to take the antibiotic with the cold's first sniffles, to rush to surgery, and so on. Doing must be supplemented by *being* ... looking inward, examining, focusing, wondering, asking."

"Prayerfulness allows us to reach a plane of experience where illness can be experienced as a natural part of life, and where its acceptance transcends passivity. The most important lessons are that prayer works and that there is no formula, no 'one best way' to pray that everyone should follow."

"Love, empathy, and compassion somehow make it possible for the mind to transcend the limitations of the body. Love is so important in this process that it is honored by giving it a place in a natural 'law.' Our love can generate a healing fire."

Read It and Change

Unintentionally, by simply reading, I had stumbled onto a type of therapy called bibliotherapy. The idea has been around for centuries.

Bibliotherapy literally means book therapy. It's also sometimes called self-help or inspirational reading. But the notion isn't a recent trend: The ancient inscription at the library of Thebes reads, "The Healing Place of the Soul." The inscription found in the medieval Abbey Library of St. Gall, Switzerland, says "The Medicine Chest of the Soul."

In its broadest sense, bibliotherapy is defined as the use of literary work in the treatment of physical or emotional problems.

Bibliotherapy sets out to change behavior or attitudes.

When it works, bibliotherapy helps you understand yourself and environment, learn from others, or find a solution to your problems. Effective bibliotherapy results in three processes: identification, catharsis and insight.

Identification begins when you recognize your own story or experience in what you are reading. You may start to realize that you and your situation or condition isn't so different from everyone else. You don't feel so alone.

Catharsis occurs when you share and vicariously experience others' motivations and conflicts in what you're reading. As you see yourself in others' descriptions, you may gain insight into your own motives and behaviors.

Your symptoms may become less frightening when you learn others experience the same thing that you do. You may find emotional release from guilt, anger, depression or tension. You understand your connection to the whole human race.

Bibliotherapy can also help you see that there may be more than one solution to a problem, and that there is value in any experience. It can provide facts to solve a problem, and encouragement to face a situation.

Learning to Read

I have needed to learn to read just for the fun of it. At one time, I thought I was wasting time reading at all. Then I thought I was wasting time reading if I was reading just for the fun of it. Now, I've learned to do both. I can get lost in a murder mystery or romance novel.

Books have become a great uplift and resource to balance out the hassles and demands of living with chronic illness. My

"R&R&R" days are days that I read, rock and rest. I try to schedule at least one of these days a week.

Here are some book that have been great guides, prods or entertainment for me. You'll find your own books that speak specifically to you.

Additional Reading

Borysenko, Joan. *Minding the Body, Mending the Mind.* New York: Bantam Doubleday Del Pub, 1993.

Carter, Les and Frank Minrith. *The Anger Workbook.* Nashville, TN: Thomas Nelson, 1993.

Claypool, John. *Tracks of a Fellow Struggler: Living and Growing Through Grief.* Insight Press, 1995.

Cloud, Henry. *Changes That Heal: How to Understand Your Past to Ensure a Heathier Future.* Zondervan Publishing House, 1993.

Cloud, Henry and John Townsend. *Boundaries.* Zondervan Publishng House, 1999.

Cloud, Henry and John Townsend. *Safe People: How to Find Relationships that Are Good for You and Avoid Those That Aren't.* Zondervan Publishing House, 1995.

Cloud, Henry and John Townsend. *12 "Christian" Beliefs That Can Drive You Crazy: Relief From False Assumptions.* Zondervan Publishing House, 1995.

Diets, Bob. *Life After Loss.* Tucson, AZ: Fisher Books, 1992.

Dossey, MD Larry. *Healing Words: The Power of Prayer and the Practice of Medicine.* San Francisco: Harper, 1997.

Dossey, MD Larry. *Prayer Is Good Medicine.* New York: HarperCollins, 1997.

Dossey, MD Larry. *The Power of Meditation and Prayer.*

Carlsbad, CA: Hay House, 1997.

Dyer, Wayne W. *Your Erroneous Zones*. Mass Market Paperback, 1997.

Ellis, Albert. *How to Live With a Neurotic*. North Hollywood, CA: Wilshire Book Co, 1986.

Frankl, Victor. *Man's Search for Ultimate Meaning*. New York: Washington Square Press, 1998.

Frankl, Victor. *The Unheard Cry for Meaning*. New York: Washington Square Press, 1997.

Girdano, Daniel and George Everly. *Controlling Stress and Tension: A Holistic Approach*. Allyn & Bacon, 1996.

Hay, Louise. *You Can Heal Your Life/101*. Carlsbad, CA: Hay House, 1987.

Hogan, Sean. *Coping with Depression in Chronic Illness*. Atlanta: Lupus Foundation of America. 800/800-4532.

Kushner, Harold S. *When Bad Things Happen to Good People*. New York: Avon, 1997.

Lerner, Harriet. *The Dance of Anger, A Woman's Guide to Changing Patterns of Intimate Relationships*. New York: Harper Collins, 1989.

Lerner, Harriet. *The Dance of Intimacy, A Woman's Guide to Courageous Acts of Change in Key Relationships*. New York: Harper Collins, 1990.

Linn, Dennis and Matthew Linn. *Healing Life's Hurts: Healing Memories Through Five Stages of Forgiveness*. Mahwah, NJ: Paulist Press, 1988.

Lorig, Kate. *Living A Healthy Life with Chronic Conditions*. Palo Alto, CA: Bull Publishing, 1994.

Peter McWilliams. *You Can't Afford the Luxury of a Negative Thought*. Los Angeles, CA: Prelude Press, 1995.

Minrith, MD, Frank B and Paul D Mier, MD. *Happiness is a Choice: The Symptoms, Causes, and Cures of Depression.* Grand Rapids, MI: Baker Book House, 1994.

Minrith, MD, Frank B and Paul D Mier, MD. *Love is a Choice: Recovery form Codependent Relationships.* Nashville, TN: Thomas Nelson, 1996.

Minrith, MD, Frank B and Paul D Mier, MD. *Love is a Choice Workbook.* Nashville, TN: Thomas Nelson, 1991.

Moyers, Bill. *Healing and the Mind.* New York: Doubleday, 1993.

Parrino, PhD, John J. *From Panic to Power: The Positive Uses of Stress.* Performance Management Pub/Aubrey Daniels, 1991.

Powell, John. *Fully Human, Fully Alive: A New Life Through a New Vision.* Allen, TX: Thomas More Press, 1989.

Powell, John. *Why Am I Afraid to Tell You Who I Am?* Tabor Publishing, 1995.

Powell, John. *Unconditional Love.* Allen, TX: Thomas More Press, 1989.

Rupp, Joyce. *Praying Our Goodbyes.* Ivey Books, 1992.

Seigle, MD, Bernie S. *Love, Medicine, and Miracles: Lessons Learned About Self-Healing from a Surgeon's Experience and Exceptional Patients.* New York: Harperperennial Library, 1990.

Simonton, MD, O. Carl and Reid Henson. *Getting Well Again.* New York: Bantam, 1992

Sobel, David S and Robert Ornstein. *The Healthy Mind Healthy Body Handbook.* ISHK Book Service, 1997.

Tada, Joni Eareckson. *Joni: An Unforgetable Story.* Zondervan Publishing House, 1997.

Viorst, Judith. *Necessary Losses.* Fireside, 1998.

Viscott, David. *Risking.* Audio Cassette, Audio Renaissance, 1989.

Wright, Beatrice A. *Physical Disability: A Psychological Approach.* Reading, MA: Addison Wesley, 1983.

Wright, Linda Raney. *Good Days Bad Days: Living with Chronic Pain and Illness.* Nashville, TN: Thomas Nelson, 1991.

Wright, Lorraine; Wendy L. Watson; and Janice Bell. *Beliefs: The Heart of Healing in Families and Illness.* New York: Basic Books, 1996.

PART V
Celebrating Life

CHAPTER 31

Living Creatively with Chronic Illness

When I was diagnosed with chronic illness, I underwent a metamorphosis. Actually, there were many metamorphoses: I went from being a caregiver to the one receiving care; from a health-care professional to a patient; from a wage earner to a disability recipient; from a robust outdoorswoman to a delicate, sun-sensitive creature; and from a "do-er" to a "be-er."

I needed patience and bulldog tenacity to redefine myself as a person with limitations and weaknesses as well as strengths and potential. After a long mourning period, I began accepting the fact that my old life was behind me. I began to slowly find ways to cope with – and even celebrate – my new life.

Finding My Place in the Sun

In order to venture back out in the world again, I had to deal with some physical problems. Ultraviolet (UV) rays, from the sun or fluorescent lighting, can aggravate lupus. I discovered I was among the lupus patients who are extremely sensitive to UV rays and possibly other sources of light, such as infrared.

I educated myself about and experimented with sunscreens to see which ones worked best for me. I learned to put them on all sun-exposed surfaces when I first got up all year long. Despite my sensitivity, I found I didn't have to go without a tan in the summer: I mastered the technique of getting natural-looking bronzed skin out of a bottle.

I also found that opaque makeup not only covered facial rashes or discoloration, but also gave further protection by blocking UV rays. I'd never worn much makeup before, and along with the light protection, it gave me a more sophisticated look. A corrective cosmetics specialist showed me how to contour my face with blush to play down my chipmunk cheeks, a side effect of steroid medication. My face was round enough to begin with.

Eye makeup presented an especially difficult challenge. Because of Sjögrens syndrome, I needed eye drops hourly. I'd put on makeup, only to wash it off with eye drops. I finally found waterproof makeup, blush, eyeliner and mascara. I carry emergency makeup supplies for repairs. Practice also made me a pro at putting in eye drops.

Long sleeves provided another shield against the sun. I would wear a loose, coordinating long-sleeved shirt over tank tops, T-shirts, short-sleeved shirts or dresses to get ventilation and UV-ray protection all summer.

In fact, it was fun to mix and match clothes to create new outfits. My new health needs also provided a great excuse to get some new clothes.

I began wearing hats to block UV rays. At first I hated them. When I was growing up, I fought my mother's attempts to make me a "little lady" by trying to get me to wear hats. I'd shove the hats to the back of the closet so they'd get crushed. I didn't want to be a "little lady." I was a tomboy who could slug it out with the best of the boys.

Having to wear a hat dug up all those old battles, and dashed my childhood images of myself as being hale and hardy. Donning a hat called a lot of attention to me.

Few people are aware that I wear hats for health reasons. It initially was not a fashion choice! When I am complimented on the way hats make me look, there is no graceful way to explain why I am wearing them. At times, I feel trapped by other people's misconceptions that I can't address without appearing negative.

Now I wear hats with a vengeance! I read somewhere that wearing a hat was just one part of dressing to kill. And I have to admit, the effect hats have on men is amazing. When I am wearing a hat, men open doors for me and offer compliments that they never would otherwise!

I Just Lost My Hair and I Can't Do a Thing with It

My hair was yet another battlefront. Illness and medications had made my already-thin and fine hair even thinner. Before my illness, I dyed my fine hair to give it extra body and reproduce the color of my hair growing up. Besides, blondes do have more fun!

Lupus, however, can make you sensitive to the caustic chemicals in permanents and dyes, stirring up disease activity and making hair fall out even more. Although hats provided UV protection, they also squashed my hair down, cut off circulation and ventilation to the scalp and further added to my hair loss.

I let my beautiful, bottle-blond hair grow out to its natural color. My sons had never seen me with anything but blond hair. We were all amazed to find my hair had become a much darker brown than it was before I started dying it.

I was accustomed to wearing my hair shoulder-length, in natural waves. With my hair falling out and becoming wispy, I cut it short and at times wore a wig. Back then, the quality of wigs within my price range were very uncomfortable and hot – not so now. Scarves and turbans also helped.

Little by little, I learned how to style my hair to accommodate my needs, my features and my hair loss. From necessity, I learned how to cut my hair myself. Not many hair stylists will listen to what you tell them, and when you do find one, she (or he) moves away!

Later, I learned that part of my hair loss may be genetic. Using monoxadil has helped. Sometimes I've toyed with the idea of shaving my head, as balding men often do. It's a sexy look.

Baubles and Bangles and Beads

Having to give up cherished rings, watches and bracelets because of swelling, joint pain or rashes was bad enough. But being forced to wear gaudy, tacky medical alert jewelry added insult to injury. Once again, it seemed circumstances were forcing more focus on my illness.

After suffering through horrible medical alert jewelry, I eventually found some fashionable, attractive 14-carat gold medical alert bracelets and necklaces. Today, designer-quality pieces are available.

A watch with an adjustable band accommodated my wrist swelling. I found pendant and ring watches for those times when rashes would break out on my wrist, or when I'd need to wear my wrist splints. I've also figured out how to attach my watch to the outside of a wrist splint.

I moved to bigger ring sizes that would slip over and not constrict swollen fingers or joints. Wide bands kept them from sliding off my fingers when the swelling subsided. There are also adjustable rings for changing finger sizes and adjustable ring guards.

When I couldn't wear my wedding and engagement rings anymore, I had new wedding rings made for my husband and me by combining gold and diamonds from several sources. Since our divorce, I've had the gold and diamonds from my ring fashioned into a cross for a necklace: to me the greatest expression of love.

Collaring Yourself

Oddly enough, the first thing about my condition that I found I could joke about was my cervical collar. Unlike my outwardly invisible illness, it was easy to spot and attracted a lot of attention.

I put the collar on in the exam room at my doctor's office and walked out into the hall. One of the nurses I knew asked what had happened to me. Without thinking, I blurted out, "This is my clerical collar ... I'm an ordained idiot!" It was great!

That led to a whole routine I could go into when asked about the collar. When asked if I'd been in a wreck or accident, I'd say, "No! *I'm* a wreck!

I began to experiment with ways to dress up my collar. At first, I attached pins and sewed on butterfly patches. Then I graduated to using turtlenecks and scarves in innovative, attractive ways.

Some people didn't even know I was wearing a neck brace

unless I told them. I have put outfits together that look more stunning with the collar and its appendages than without it.

Wearing a vest, sweater or jacket with pleated skirts or slacks made my lumbar support brace barely noticeable. It actually seemed to serve as a kind of girdle and made me look thinner.

Skirts and slacks that require a belt helped hold the brace in place and kept it from riding up. The brace can be hot, so it was important to wear cotton fabrics that could breathe in summer.

Now that I've traded in the cervical collar and lumbar support for wrist, ankle, knee and finger splints, I try to find attractive, colorful models. Fortunately, long skirts are fashionable now. Like slacks, they cover leg supports well. I can look sporty and supported at the same time!

The Masked Wonder

At one point, when I was on daily chemotherapy for 18 months for kidney involvement, I needed to wear a black "rebreather" contoured facemask anytime I went out of the house. It protected me from life-threatening infections.

People at ATM machines would think I was going to rob them. Mothers would grab their children in the grocery store and run from me. Babies would cry. The reactions I was getting made me want to go back home, curl up and die.

I finally had a good cry and talk with myself. I came to the decision I'd just have to get over it and get on with life. No one else could run my errands for me. I began to try to think of ways to have fun with my black mask.

I put butterfly stickers and pins on the mask, along with heart and flower stickers. I even had a pin made that said "I'm looking for Zorro."

I now wear a personal air purifier around my neck that helps with infection. I dress it up with scarves and bandannas. People think it's my pager. I found that something abhorrent can be made manageable by being creative and having fun with it.

Feet Don't Fail Me Now

No matter how you try to get around it, orthopedic shoes are a nightmare. The color and style selection is the pits! They look like the latest Pentagon project and cost about as much.

You'll be sorely tested to find something that looks good with skirts, and it's next to impossible to find dress shoes. High heels are definitely out if you have any back or lower-body joint problems.

You can now find some pretty fashionable walking shoes. They look better and still give the support that you need. Once again, it may take stubbornness to keep looking for what your feet need. A combination of shoes and orthotic devices could help give you the desired look and meet your medical requirements.

Sizing It Up ... and Down

As my disease fluctuates, and with medications that add or subtract pounds, my weight gains and losses become yet another wardrobe challenge. I now have clothes in three sizes to accommodate weight swings.

Elastic waistbands, loose cover-ups, vertical and horizontal stripes, jackets, vests – all are weapons in my arsenal for dressing to kill. When the size of my waist and hips fluctuates, I can feel good about how I'm dressed without going out and buying a whole new wardrobe.

The harder struggle is against our society's mandate to be

thin. It's sometimes difficult to remember that I am sexy, smart and worthy, regardless of my weight and clothing size. My "greatness" is determined by what's inside anyway!

The Internal Makeover

Unless I have come to love myself just as I am, looking polished or sophisticated on the outside makes no difference on the inside. On the other hand, I can look great and feel good about myself even if I still feel rotten physically.

There is a very delicate balancing act between using my appearance to cover up or deny my illness and accepting my illness as just another part of who I am. Chronic illness can assault my self-image, displacing my identity and sense of worthiness.

In reaching acceptance, I can use my appearance as a total expression of who I am ... my total personhood, illness and all. Trying to forget, cover up or "pass" as normal is the best way to focus on my illness and drain my energy with performance anxiety.

If I feel good about myself, that will show through any makeup or wardrobe. Likewise, if I don't feel good about myself, no amount of effort can cover that up. I try to let my external appearance reflect my internal wardrobe of acceptance, joy, peace and love, and not just be a cover up for what I don't want other people to see.

Putting It All Together

Every ending is a new beginning. Though you may have little choice in your circumstances, you still retain the freedom to choose your attitude in those circumstances! It's mind over matter: If you don't mind, it doesn't matter!

An attitude of love and self-acceptance allows me to emerge from my chrysalis as a thing of beauty, like a bright-winged butterfly. That attitude frees me to be more than my illness, more than what I look like.

I have seen many people who cling to "before"-illness pictures of themselves, and hide "after" photos. They recognize themselves only in their former lives. I rather like my "after" pictures now. That is who I have become.

The way I look is ultimately determined by what inner light shines from within. Makeup, clothing and jewelry only enhance beauty – they can't create it!

CHAPTER 32

The Mind/Body/Spirit Connection

Volumes have been written about the mind's influence on the body's natural healing abilities. In learning to live with lupus and many other rheumatic diseases over many years, I have been experiencing what modern science is finding out about the mind/body connection.

I have also begun to discover what the additional component of spirit can add to the mind/body connection. For me, all three levels affect wholeness, balance and healing.

Before the modern era of medical technology, healers knew that the mind, body and spirit were intimately and intricately interwoven. The role of healers of old was to help the "diseased" person find and tap into those inner healing potentials.

Our scientific age has taken the focus and responsibility away from the individual and assigned all the power of healing to medical technology, paternalistic practitioners and institutions.

Sometimes patients are treated like children, as if they don't have minds or wisdom of their own. Of course, modern medicine can boast many miracles, but it is still limited.

The book *The Healing Journey* by O. Carl Simonton, MD, and Reid Henson (see "Reading Therapy," Chapter 30) examines a personal spiritual experience, healing, and the finite knowledge of medical science. *Healing Words* by Larry Dossey, MD, also deals with the spiritual component of healing.

Nourishing your spirit can facilitate healing in a way that science will never be able to understand or duplicate. After all, no matter how much knowledge health-care professionals accrue, they will still be "practicing" medicine.

The real medicine resides in delving into your own personal well of wisdom and healing. If you keep searching, eventually you'll tap into the much larger and deeper river of wisdom and healing that flows through the ages. It's the same wisdom, no matter how you reach it. Until you make that effort, attempts at healing will only be marginal, fragmented and momentary.

My spiritual path is Christianity. I enhance my spirituality with meditation and other practices. My goal is to find a spiritual connection with God as I understand Him that awakens my spirit.

Your spiritual path may take a well-trodden route: Christianity, Judaism, Buddhism, Taoism, Islam or another organized religion. Some may find spiritual comfort from contemplation and yoga, or experience what the poet Emily Dickinson referred to as awe and circumference through a reverence for nature. Others will find that spiritual connection elsewhere, or from a mixture of influences. How you travel is less important than undertaking the journey.

Breaking the Mind/Body Feedback Loop

Breath Prayers

Stress doesn't happen just in the mind. Stress engages every system of the body. In several of the previous chapters, we've discussed how stress influences the body, often translating into worsened symptoms, which then produces more stress. We've also discussed how unresolved emotional issues can cause or worsen stress, as well as physical and psychological methods for dealing with them.

You can also break this unhealthy mind/body feedback loop by spiritual means. After years of looking for ways to approach life in a healthy way, I learned to combine several techniques into one method, which I call breath prayers. They've become a powerful force in my journey with chronic illness. With them, I find I can spiritually transcend my circumstances.

Breath prayers' techniques combine many proven psychodynamic approaches to health with a spiritual element. They offer meditation and deep muscle relaxation, breathing exercises and affirmations. They fit in with such methods as thought-stopping, distraction therapy and anxiety management training.

Here's how I do them: I take an affirmation that connects my spirit to my higher spirit as a prayer, and repeat it as I exhale in a "perfect breath." This yoga breathing technique that harmonizes mind and body involves inhaling and exhaling in a one-to-two ratio. Inhale through the nose counting to three. Hold the breath as long as it's comfortable. Exhale through the mouth to a count of six. Use the abdominal muscles to pull the breath deep down into the gut. Once again, hold the breath as long as it is comfortable.

The affirmation needs to be about seven syllables – give or

take a few syllables – to fit comfortably in the exhalation of a perfect breath. Repeat the affirmation every time you exhale.

For me, the most meaningful affirmations are found in the Bible. You may find meaningful spiritual affirmations in your own inspirational reading. You may also want to look in the many books of spiritual affirmations now offered in libraries and bookstores. Many of them are specifically aimed at certain segments of the population, such as businesspeople, mothers, African-Americans.

Affirmations probably first came into wide usage with 12-step programs, such as Alcoholics Anonymous, to help people cope with their problems one day at a time. Many also offer wisdom to people with chronic illness.

The affirmation needs to fit your situation like a glove. When I find the right spiritual affirmation, I actually feel a mind, body, spirit recognition reflex on a cellular level ... an "AHA!"

Here are some of the breath prayers that I use most regularly:

"In my weakness is Your strength" (II Corinthians 12:9).
"You heal all my dis-eases" (Psalm 103:3).
"You try and know my anxious thoughts" (Psalm 139:23).
"Your perfect love casts out my fear" (1 John 4:18).

If you aren't comfortable with these biblical breath prayers, adapt other proverbs or prayers or sacred text from your own source of spirituality. For me, breath prayers are most effective when they follow this simple formula: Each affirmation directly addresses your Higher Power with "You" and claims a promise in the present tense.

Your Higher Power may be the universe, the earth, Brahma,

Allah or Yahweh. A Buddhist's breath prayer might be "You take me through life to my next life." A Hindu's breath prayer could take the form of "You help me break free of this world."

Muslims might contemplate some form of the saying, "You give me life, death and rebirth." Sikhs might utter, "You give me religious tolerance." The most important points are that your spirit connects with your Higher Spirit, and you affirm your belief system.

I use breath prayers as my mantra for a period of anywhere from 20 to 60 minutes of deep relaxation and meditation a day. It trains my mind, body and spirit to relax, and gives me a positive, conditioned reflex. After that, my mind, body and spirit are trained to relax at the signal of the breath prayer no matter where I am or what I am doing.

I repeat this breath prayer on waking, throughout the day and when falling asleep that night, on the exhaling of each breath. The unconscious mind is most accessible to the conscious mind when falling asleep, on waking and during deep meditative relaxation. Repeating breath prayers during these times will help replace obsessive negative thoughts, and rewrite the unhealthy scripts of my unconscious mind. It's a mind/body/spirit workout!

Strengthening Your Spirit

Once after surgery, my disease activity kicked up. I was thrown into intense, debilitating chest pain. Curled up on my bed, I began repeating the breath prayer, "I'm healed in Your presence" as I exhaled over and over and over.

The pain became more and more intense. It scared me, but I kept on saying the breath prayer. The "perfect breaths" and the positive scripture calmed me. Eventually, I dropped off to sleep. The pain was gone the next morning. That was just one of many times breath prayers helped relieve my pain, bring healing and soothed me when I would have been distraught.

I've found release and healing by giving all of my experience to my God as I experience Him. Sometimes I may think I need physical healing when in fact my broken heart or wounded spirit needs healing more.

The beneficial effects of breath prayers are cumulative and additive. The more I use them, the more powerful and transforming they become! Part of their power comes from sharing them with others.

In that sharing, I focus on the victories – not on what healing remains to be done. As a medical professional, this is a real challenge. My training focuses me on illness.

I transcend my mental and physical limits to find victories and miracles moment to moment. Breath prayers keep my mind focused on my spirit and its connection to every other living thing, and to the power beyond this life.

Breath prayers, like meditating, quiet the mind's endless, useless chatter. Shutting up these nonproductive ramblings allows my body to relax, blot out pain and regenerate. Breath prayers turn off my mind's static and allow my body to heal, working alongside my antibiotics and anti-inflammatory drugs.

Love

Love is a powerful healing force. Whatever your spiritual path, you will be able to find affirmations about love for breath prayers. "May Your love flow through me," a verse from the New Testament, is my most frequent and fervent breath prayer.

This verse reminds me of love's greatest lessons, which are to love freely, without expectation of reward or return, and to allow the object of your love to be him or herself. All are part of the Higher Spirit's larger plan. Examine your own philosophy about love and its healing benefits to find some breath prayers that fit you.

I am learning about breath prayers by using them in the laboratory of everyday living. With them, I am finding healing, happiness, transcendence and balance that I have never found before. It's an ever-evolving learning process that will last as long as I live.

If you want to know more about breath prayers, you may also want to read my book or listen to my tape, *Prayer Without Ceasing: Breath Prayers* (Vital Issue Press, 1998). Write to Celebrate Life, 1651 Northlake Springs Ct, Decatur, GA 30033.

CHAPTER 33

Taking Flight

In the first eight years after I was diagnosed with chronic illness, I struggled to find a way to live, and not just survive. Just about the time I thought I'd rebuilt my life, my marriage fell apart.

Dealing with each crisis as it presented itself was all I could manage. Every day I made it through was a victory. I concentrated on putting one foot in front of the other. Paying my bills, getting food on the table and taking care of my sons and myself took every ounce of energy I could muster.

Somewhere along the way, as I struggled with the present, I lost the ability to envision my own future.

The Arthritis Foundation began developing a self-help course for people with lupus. I got involved. One exercise asked you to list things that you loved to do. You rated when you last did them and were encouraged to dream up some outrageous things you might want to do.

I suddenly realized I had no dreams.

In my old life, I'd had hopes and goals for my marriage, my family and my career. All that had changed. Some days, my big goal was to sit up for a few hours.

Just realizing that I could and needed to dream again got me started.

Over the next few years, I started paying special attention to a TV commercial. Grand, sweeping music would accompany a scenic vista of beautiful Lookout Mountain in Chattanooga. In the next few seconds, someone wearing a huge, multicolored set of wings – a hang glider – would jump off, and begin a silent, graceful descent.

My spirit would jump inside of me and say "Wow!" Finally, while teaching one of the self-help workshop meetings, during the Things I Love to Do exercise, I wrote down hang gliding.

I'd never really done it. But the seed of thought was planted and a dream began growing.

Whenever I'd hear the music starting, I'd run to the TV and watch in wonder like a child. The thought of jumping off a mountain scared me to death. But something kept pulling me.

I watched the commercial for a year before I made the first phone call. Maybe I was afraid to have my hopes dashed, but finally, I had to see what would be involved if I ... *really did this thing*.

I asked what provisions were made for the physically challenged, and how physically fit I needed to be. I found out I needed to be able to run only a few steps for takeoff. A "pilot" would go up with me.

I knew I could do that. The next task was to work toward making my dream become a reality.

I began using the four P's ... pacing, prioritizing, planning and problem solving. I was P-ing all over the place. In June, I set Labor Day weekend as my target date.

If this was going to work at all, I had to be brutally honest with myself about my abilities. No one else would be there to help. Other than the pilot, this was going to be a solo flight from start to finish – I was sad no one was around to share it with me, but I wasn't going to let that keep me from doing it.

I would need plenty of rest for all the driving and physical stress. The hang-gliding group told me I should be prepared for imperfect weather conditions – I might be told to come back the next day. I figured I needed a motel room in case there was a delay and I had to stay near Lookout Mountain. My AAA motel book listed a place that was fairly close and reasonably priced.

After the flight, I knew I would need plenty of rest before driving home, so friends who lived on Signal Mountain, one mountain over, agreed to let me crash at their house.

I also knew I needed to limit the outing to a maximum of a few days. Being outside the filtered air of my home increased my risk of getting serious, life-threatening sinus infections.

Dryness from Sjögrens syndrome has made me susceptible to these infections, some of which have lasted over a year. Other infections have settled in next to the carotid artery. Some have required surgery; at times I've required intravenous antibiotics to fight them. They aren't anything to play around with.

After a month of thought, I called the hang gliding place in July to make an appointment for the Saturday of Labor Day weekend, two months away. I cleared my calendar on either side of the big event to be able to rest before and after the flight.

Most people thought I was crazy for even thinking about doing this. I began asking people to pray for me.

At one time, the two-hour drive alone would have put me into a tremendous tailspin and flare for weeks or months. Here I was planning the drive, hang gliding and visiting friends.

I stepped up my exercise regimen just a hair to try to increase my physical fitness. The enterprise began taking on some kind of spiritual element that I really can't completely describe.

The closer the actual event came, the more the whole experience seemed beyond my wildest dreams. Doubts and fears would surface. I'd do everything I could to fight them: meditation, relaxation, breath prayers. I wrote about my doubts and fears. And I imagined myself every step of the way: preparing, driving, running a few steps ... and flying.

My doctor guided me on how and whether to increase medications for pain and disease activity. She also recommended splints to reinforce my wrists and ankles.

There were other preparations: My car needed a checkup to handle the trip. Beamer, my wonderful dog-friend, needed someone to care for him. I stocked up on groceries and filled prescriptions well in advance so that when I got home I wouldn't have to go back out for a while.

I assembled an outfit that would protect me from the sun's ultraviolet rays. More importantly, the outfit – including splints and hat – needed to be color-coordinated and stylish.

Even if I was feeling sick, I didn't want it to be obvious. I was determined to look good even if I didn't feel good.

As the big day approached, I began developing a significant sinus infection. All conventional and rational wisdom would have dictated that I call off the trip, go to the doctor, take antibiotics and go to bed. But a conversation with my Higher Spirit and myself convinced me that that route led to stifled energy, and endings.

The thought of going ahead with my plan filled my spirit with energy, life, light and joy. I found peace with my decision only on the morning I was to leave. Against all reason, I decided to take the leap of faith, taking one task and step at a time ... getting up, taking medicine, eating, dressing.

I gave myself permission to say "Uncle" at any point and call it all off. I stumbled into the car and pointed it north. I'd given myself plenty of time in case I got lost. I didn't need any extra stress.

I celebrated each exit and city that I passed rather than focusing on how much farther I had to drive. I took frequent breaks to stretch muscles and joints.

I'd even chair-dance in the driver's seat to the special uplifting music that I'd taped for the trip. Moving around kept my circulation going and prevented stiffness and stress on joints. People behind me thought I was crazy. Truck drivers blew their horns and cheered me on.

I finally found myself on top of Lookout Mountain, fighting to find a parking space on the edge of the road that bordered a cliff. The parking lot was filled with dozens of bright, colorful hang gliders positioned for takeoff. People milled around, petted their dogs, ate and sipped drinks.

When I went inside, I found that the wind and weather conditions weren't just right for take off. People were really backed up waiting for their turns. Most of the pilots were on the ground in a field below. The ground crew put me on the waiting list and said they'd call me when it was my time.

The afternoon passed as I looked at the beauty and majesty of the mountain, the sheer cliff and drop, the beautiful green pasture and the ever-changing cloud formations letting glints of sunshine and sky through.

A few people were able to take flight when there were rare windows of opportunity. Their flights were beautiful but brief ... 45 to 60 seconds to the bottom.

Finally, the crew sent me down to the pasture below, saying I might have a better chance to get a flight by being pulled off by an airplane. From down below I was able to watch a few people do loop-de-loops to prolong their flights. They'd get to the bottom, collect their gear and wait again for another window.

As the sun began to get low in the sky, I was told to come back the next morning. I tottered back to my car and slowly found my way across the spine of the mountain to my motel.

My room was truly rustic – really more like a cabin. There was no TV or phone. With my music playing full blast, I wrote in my journal and sang along with my tapes. A long tub soak was essential for sore, stiff joints and muscles.

I went to bed early and woke up the next morning to a hazy, hot day.

I gulped down my medication, along with fruit bars and dried fruit I'd brought. I couldn't spend my precious resources of energy and money on going out and finding breakfast.

So far, so good. I'd done a pretty decent job up to this point of balancing my perceived demands of the trip with my perceived resources.

The weather was still a difficulty when I reached the field. A couple of people were ahead of me. The airplane that would pull me skyward looked more like a bicycle.

Finally, by early afternoon, the clouds broke and the wind settled. It was my turn. My nervousness turned into sheer wonder and excitement as I got into my harness on top of the pilot's back.

Pulled by the plane, we took off and started climbing, circling the field. All I could say over and over was "OH! MY GOD! OH! MY GOD!" I'm sure the pilot thought I was a complete idiot. We swept by the mountain cliff, where other flyers were waiting for their turn.

As we reached about 3,000 feet, the plane circled and let us go. We were on our own to navigate the wind back down to the pasture.

Silently, we glided above the hawks and eagles. Our eyeglasses misted as we swept through a cloud. We sailed by the takeoff cliff a couple more times. People waved and cheered ... if they only knew!

Cows looked like ants, houses were matchboxes and the expanse of clouds was unbelievable. We floated above Lookout Mountain, where I'd gone on my honeymoon.

I'd broken the bonds of earth. Something about the journey seemed to sum up my life up to that point. The feeling of transcendence encouraged me to face whatever difficulties lay ahead, and to strive to achieve greater heights.

The flight lasted 30 minutes. The pilot said it was the longest and best flight he'd had all summer. It was like a hand was holding us up there.

Despite my awe and excitement, I was terribly nauseated as we landed. I later learned that my eardrum had ruptured during the flight. I smiled, choked back the feeling of nausea, and stumbled to my car, saying as little as I could. I was afraid to open my mouth.

With a Coke in hand to calm my stomach, almost in a trance, I headed to my friends' house. What had seemed impossible had become reality. I called them on the car phone, shouting, "I did it! I did it! Get the couch ready!"

My friends were all waiting in the front yard when I arrived. I excitedly babbled every detail of the flight. They were awestruck, and full of congratulations. They helped me to the couch, where they waited on me hand and foot for the rest of the evening. I drove home the next day.

A week or so later, pictures arrived. The pilot had taken them from a camera on the wing. Just looking at them filled me with joy and reverence. Even today, just thinking about the experience gives me a thrill.

I paid a big price physically, but it was worth it. Following my heart's passion made me feel more alive and well than I ever would have if I'd stayed at home in bed.

Of course, I was only able to make my dream a reality by acknowledging that I was no longer my former self. I wasn't able to hang glide the way I might have been able to before illness. I did it the best way I could. I found new, creative ways that accommodated my limits and potentials, strengths and weaknesses.

The trip would never have happened if I'd thought, "If I can't do it the way I used to, I won't do it at all." Instead, I thought, "I'll do what I can, when I can, as I am able."

I reinvented myself as a new person, to escape the bonds of earth, and of illness. Like the butterfly, I had to undergo a complete metamorphosis to take flight.

The growth of the caterpillar, which is considered just another form of the butterfly, isn't gradual or continuous. Sudden growth spurts follow periods of no change and growth.

Eventually the caterpillar sheds its stretched-to-the-limit skin, and reveals a new layer that will accommodate its growth.

When the caterpillar is full-grown, it transforms into a chrysalis, where it neither eats nor moves about. Inside, the caterpillar's body breaks down. Imaginal disks in the chrysalis direct the total reorganization of the caterpillar's body into a butterfly.

The butterfly's struggle to free itself from the chrysalis pumps blood into the wings so they stretch and harden. Only then is the butterfly ready for flight.

In the life cycle of the butterfly, the function of the caterpillar is nutrition, the chrysalis is structural reorganization, and the butterfly is reproduction.

I feel the grief process I went through with chronic illness parallels the life cycle of the butterfly. I get stuck and resist stages of breaking down, reorganizing and restructuring.

I still grieve, but it's not so bad any more. I move through the grief quicker and pay a smaller price. With the help of the Spirit, my ultimate goal is to become more than my illness. That's when I can transcend the experience, and fly.

In my den, a painting by a friend's young son hangs over the mantle. In it, a hang glider flies over the mountains in Italy. A small, solitary figure soars toward a dark cloudbank, with the sun streaming in from crevices in the cloud. Somehow, it feels as though that picture represents me.

Appendix A – Relaxation Techniques

BENSON'S RELAXATION TECHNIQUE

The relaxation response is a natural protective mechanism that allows us to turn off harmful effects from stress. This response decreases heart rate, lowers metabolism, slows breathing, and brings the body back into a healthier balance.

Four basic elements evoke Benson's relaxation response:
1. A quiet environment

2. An object to dwell upon

3. A passive attitude

4. A comfortable position

In order to trigger the relaxation response, follow the steps below:
1. Sit quietly in a comfortable position.

2. Close your eyes.

3. Deeply relax all your muscles, beginning at your feet and progressing up to your face. Keep them relaxed.

4. Breathe through your nose. Become aware of your breathing. As you breathe out, say the word "one" silently to yourself. Breathe easily and naturally.

5. Continue for 10 to 20 minutes. You may open your eyes to check the time, but do not use an alarm. When you finish, sit quietly for several minutes, at first with your eyes closed and later with your eyes opened. Do not stand up for a few minutes.

Do not worry about whether you are successful in achieving a deep level of relaxation. Maintain a passive attitude and permit relaxation to occur at its own pace. When distracting thoughts occur, merely return to repeating "one." With practice, the response should come with little effort. Practice the technique once or twice daily, but not within two hours after any meal since the digestive process seems to interfere with the elicitation of the relaxation response.

Both of the following muscle relaxation methods have been used with permission of Kenneth B. Matheny, Ph.D., of Georgia State University. At first it is easiest for someone to read the steps to you as you perform the techniques. Or you may want to read the instructions into a tape recorder with relaxing music or nature sounds in the background.

MUSCLE RELAXATION METHOD ONE

You should be in a comfortable and quiet environment: sitting in a chair, or on a piece of furniture that allows you to stretch your legs out. If you can concentrate for 20 minutes without falling asleep, you may lie down on a bed, sofa or even the floor. It is important for you to complete the relaxation instructions without falling asleep to obtain maximum benefit from the technique. If you wish, you may sleep after the instructions are completed.

Loosen any tight clothing that you may be wearing, like a tie or belt, and if your shoes are uncomfortable, take them off. You are now ready to begin the relaxation technique. You will relax your toes first and then progressively move up to and relax each part of the body until you finish with the face.

1. Close your eyes and concentrate on your toes: Curl them down toward the soles of your feet and tense them vigorously – hold that tension for about five seconds. People with rheumatoid arthritis or fibromyalgia need to tense gently. As you count to five, you should tense the toes more and more vigorously. 1 – 2 – 3 – tighter – 4 – a little tighter – 5. Before letting the tension go, take a deep breath. Let the breath out and release the tension in your toes at the same time. Notice the feeling of relief. Then repeat the word "relax" to yourself. "Relax. Relax. Relax."

2. With your eyes closed, now concentrate on your calves, the lower part of your legs: Point your toes up toward your face and tighten your calves vigorously. Hold that tension for about 5 seconds. As you count to 5, you should tense the calves tighter and tighter. 1 – 2 – 3 – tighter – 4 – a little tighter – 5. Take a deep breath and let go of the tension in your calves and your breath at the same time. Repeat the word "relax" to yourself. "Relax. Relax. Relax."

3. Concentrate on your thighs, the upper part of your legs: Extend your legs out in front of you and point the toes up toward your face once again, this time tightening your thighs vigorously. Hold that tension for about 5 seconds. As you count to 5, you should tense the thighs more and more vigorously.

1 – 2 – 3 – tighter – 4 – a little tighter – 5. Take a deep breath, and then let go of the tension in your thighs and the deep breath at the same time. Good. Repeat the word "relax" to yourself. "Relax. Relax. Relax."

Notice the difference now between the feelings that you are getting from your legs as compared to the feelings from your upper body. Your legs are more relaxed and heavier, and you may be feeling a tingling sensation from them. Your upper body is tighter. Concentrate on the difference for a moment.

4. Now, concentrate on your buttocks: Tense them by pushing this part of your body down against the seat of your chair or against the bed or sofa. Push down. 1 – 2 – 3 – tighter – 4 – a little tighter – 5. Take a deep breath, and let go of the tension in your buttocks and the deep breath at the same time. Good. Repeat the word "relax" to yourself. "Relax. Relax. Relax."

5. Concentrate on your abdomen: Tense this part of your body by imagining that you are going to protect yourself from a punch or blow coming toward your stomach. OK, tense your abdomen. 1 – 2 – 3 – tighter – 4 – a little tighter – 5. Take a deep breath. Hold it for a second and then let go of the tension in your stomach and the breath at the same time. Very good. Repeat the word "relax" to yourself. "Relax. Relax. Relax."

6. Concentrate on your chest: Tighten your chest by clasping your hands together – the palm of one hand pressing against the palm of your other hand. Press them together. 1 – 2 – 3 – harder – 4 – a little harder – 5. Take a deep breath. Hold that for a second; and, now, let your hands go from each other very slowly. Let your breath out at the same time. Good. Repeat the word "relax" to yourself. "Relax. Relax. Relax."

7. Concentrate on your shoulders: Tighten your shoulders by shrugging them, bringing your head down between your shoulders as far as it will go. Shrug your shoulders. 1 – 2 – 3 – tighter – 4 – a little tighter – 5. Take a deep breath. Hold the breath for a second. Now slowly let go of the tension in your shoulders and let your breath out at the same time. Good. Repeat the word "relax" to yourself. "Relax. Relax. Relax."

8. Concentrate on your arms: Extend them out in front of you, tighten your fists, and tense the upper portion of your arms and your forearms together. 1 – 2 – 3 – tighter – 4 – a little tighter – 5. Take a deep breath. Now slowly let go of the tension in your arms and the breath at the same time. Repeat the word "relax" to yourself. "Relax. Relax. Relax."

9. Concentrate on your throat: Tighten your throat by pressing your chin down against the upper part of your chest. Press down vigorously. 1 – 2 – 3 – harder – 4 – a little harder – 5. Take a deep breath. Let both the tension in your throat and the breath out at the same time. Repeat the word "relax" to yourself. "Relax. Relax. Relax."

10. Concentrate on the back of your neck and head: Tense the back of your neck and head by pressing your head down against the back of your shoulders. Press hard. 1 – 2 – 3 –harder – 4 – a little harder – 5. Take a deep breath. Let the tension and breath out at the same time. Good. Repeat the word "relax" to yourself. "Relax. Relax. Relax."

11. Concentrate on your face – your forehead, eyes, nose, cheeks, mouth and chin: Tense these areas of your face by making a funny face. Wrinkle your forehead, close your eyes tightly, and grit your teeth at the same time. Tense your face. 1 – 2 – 3 – tighter – 4 – a little tighter – 5. Take a deep breath. Let the breath and tension go. Now, make another funny face: Wrinkle your forehead, open your eyes wide, and open your mouth as big as it will open. Stretch your face. 1– 2 – 3 – tighter – 4 – a little tighter – 5. Take a deep breath. Let the breath and tension go. Repeat the word "relax" to yourself. "Relax. Relax. Relax."

Notice the feedback that you are getting from your body now compared to the way it felt before. It should be more relaxed, heavier and perhaps you are feeling a tingling throughout your body.

The final step of this method is to go back and concentrate on each body part you have already muscularly relaxed. You will concentrate on each part and tell it to relax five times. You will not contract your muscles at this time but simply concentrate and think of the repetition of the word "relax." This will allow you to remove any worrisome thoughts from your response system and facilitate the state of relaxation you have already achieved.

Think of your toes — Tell them to Relax. Relax. Relax. Relax. Relax.
Think of your calves — Tell them to Relax. Relax. Relax. Relax. Relax.
Think of your thighs — Tell them to Relax. Relax. Relax. Relax. Relax.
Think of your buttocks — Tell them to Relax. Relax. Relax. Relax. Relax.
Think of your stomach — Tell it to Relax. Relax. Relax. Relax. Relax.
Think of your chest — Tell it to Relax. Relax. Relax. Relax. Relax.
Think of your shoulders — Tell them to Relax. Relax. Relax. Relax. Relax.
Think of your arms — Tell them to Relax. Relax. Relax. Relax. Relax.
Think of your throat — Tell it to Relax. Relax. Relax. Relax. Relax.

Think of the back of your neck and head — Tell them to Relax. Relax. Relax.
Relax. Relax.

Think of your face — Tell it to Relax. Relax. Relax. Relax. Relax.

MUSCLE RELAXATION METHOD TWO

Remove constraining items such as watches, rings, eyeglasses, contact lenses and shoes, if desirable. Recline in a tilt-back chair or sit upright with your feet firmly planted on the floor and arms lying loosely in your lap. Closing your eyes will often be helpful. Release tension immediately rather than gradually. Once a group of muscles is relaxed, do not move them unnecessarily.

1. Extend arms in front of yourself and clinch fists. For this and each successive muscle group, tense for seven seconds and then rest muscles for 20 - 30 seconds before moving on to the next muscle group.

2. Extend arms in front of yourself and point fingers toward the ceiling as though you are pushing a wall.

3. Touch fingers to shoulders to tense biceps.

4. Shut eyes tightly to tense muscles around the eyes, in forehead and in temples (skip this exercise if you are wearing contact lenses).

5. Push tongue against roof of mouth, clinch molar teeth, and pull corners of lips around as though trying to touch ears.

6. Pull chin down one inch from sternum (breast bone) and at the same time try to pull chin further toward sternum and backward toward your back. This sets up antagonistic muscle reaction and causes head to tremor.

7. Take a deep breath and hunch shoulders up toward ears.

8. Pull shoulders back as though trying to touch them together in the back.

9. Suck stomach in as though trying to touch backbone.

10. Push rear end into chair to tense buttock muscles.

11. Extend legs in front of yourself and lift heels six inches off floor to tense thigh muscles.

12. With legs extended and heels resting on floor, point toes toward knees to tense calf muscles.

13. With legs extended and heels resting on floor, curl toes under toward

arches (tense for only three seconds because these muscles easily experience cramps).

14. Now, review the condition of each of these muscle groups and visualize them becoming more and more relaxed. See muscle fibers becoming looser and longer — stretching out like wet spaghetti. You may notice that your palms are becoming warmer, that your upper torso is becoming heavier and heavier. Concentrate on these effects since they are evidence of deep relaxation.

Sit quietly for several moments. You might wish to use this experience for implanting more firmly in your mind certain goals that are important to you. Picture the goal clearly in your mind, and see yourself reaching your goal. Make your picture as vivid with as much detail as possible. You may find this is a great aid to your motivation.

BREATHING EXERCISE

The following technique, used by permission of Kenneth B. Matheny, Ph.D., of Georgia State University, will help to regulate your breathing and equalize your oxygen and carbon dioxide levels.

1. Sit comfortably with feet firmly planted on the floor, body weight resting evenly on the spinal column, hands resting on lap, eyes closed and garments appropriately loosened.

2. Before beginning the prescribed breathing, take your pulse. Count the beats for three seconds and double.

3. Inhale for three seconds; hold for 12 seconds; and exhale for six seconds.

4. On the sixth cycle hold your breath for 20 seconds and afterwards exhale explosively. Afterwards sit quietly for one minute while allowing your breathing to reach its own level.

5. Take your pulse for a second time while sitting quietly. If you were nervous to begin with, you will often show a lowered pulse.

Practice this exercise frequently until you can visualize the resulting relaxation before you begin. The more you practice, the better the results. You might wish to use the exercise to prepare yourself for situations that are likely to make you anxious or angry. The entire experience takes roughly 2 1/2 minutes.

Appendix B – About the Arthritis Foundation

The Arthritis Foundation is the only national, voluntary health organization that works for all people affected by any of the 100-plus forms of arthritis or related diseases. Volunteers in chapters nationwide help to support research, professional and community education programs, services for people with arthritis, government advocacy on behalf of people with arthritis, and fund-raising activities.

The American Juvenile Arthritis Organization (AJAO), a council of the Arthritis Foundation, focuses its efforts on the problems and issues related to arthritis and similar conditions in children. It is composed of children, parents, health professionals, teachers and others who are concerned specifically about juvenile arthritis.

The goal of the Arthritis Foundation is two-fold: to support research to find the cure for and prevention of arthritis, and to improve the quality of life for those affected by arthritis. Public contributions enable the Arthritis Foundation to fulfill this mission. The Arthritis Foundation is the largest non-government supporter of arthritis-related research in the United States. In fact, at least 80 cents of every dollar contributed to the Arthritis Foundation helps fund the research, programs and services that make a difference in people's lives.

Research holds the key to future cures for and preventions of arthritis, but it takes time for researchers to make substantial progress. The good news is your condition doesn't have to rob you of the activities you enjoy most until those cures are found. The Arthritis Foundation believes it is equally important to improve the quality of life for people with arthritis today, which is why chapters offer information, programs and services to communities nationwide.

The Arthritis Foundation has more than 150 offices in the United States, so your road to living successfully with arthritis may be just a phone call away. Many chapters offer services such as those described in the following sections. Check your local phone book or call 800/283-7800 to find the Arthritis Foundation chapter nearest you and learn what programs and services it offers.

Medical and Self-Care Programs

Taking care of yourself physically is an important part of living well with arthritis or a related condition. The first step in that process is to get an early and accurate diagnosis from a physician. The Arthritis Foundation chapter in your area may offer the following programs and services to help further your efforts to take care of yourself.

Physician Referral

Working with a physician who is knowledgeable about arthritis is the key to a successful treatment program. Most Arthritis Foundation offices can provide you with a list of doctors in your area who specialize in the evaluation and treatment of arthritis and arthritis-related diseases.

Exercise Programs

Regular exercise is one of the most important steps in controlling your arthritis. You don't need to work out to the point of exhaustion to benefit from exercise. Every bit of activity is good for you physically and emotionally. These exercise programs are designed specifically for people with arthritis, and are led by specially trained instructors.

Joint Efforts. This arthritis movement program teaches gentle, undemanding movement exercises to help you maintain or regain your range of motion, even if you use a walker or wheelchair. Joint Efforts can also help decrease your pain, stiffness and depression.

PACE (People with Arthritis Can Exercise). You can increase your joint flexibility and range of motion and help maintain muscle strength using the gentle activities found in the Arthritis Foundation exercise program PACE. It can help you no matter your fitness level. Two videotapes that show basic and advanced levels of the program are available from your local Arthritis Foundation chapter for preview or for practice at home.

Arthritis Foundation Aquatics Program. This water exercise program was originally co-developed by the Arthritis Foundation and the YMCA. You can increase your muscle strength and endurance with this water exercise program. The water's buoyancy allows you to exercise without straining your joints.

Educational Courses

If you live with a chronic condition like arthritis, taking an active role in your health care is especially important. Call your local Arthritis Foundation chapter to learn if the following classes are offered in your area.

Arthritis Foundation Self-Help Courses.

Gain the knowledge, skills and confidence needed to actively manage your condition. Courses focus on proper exercises, medications, relaxation techniques, pain and fatigue management, nutrition, and other relevant topics. Whether you have arthritis, fibromyalgia or lupus, one of the three different curriculums can help. Classes meet once weekly for six or seven weeks.

Bone Up On Arthritis

Learn much of the same information that is taught in Arthritis Foundation Self-Help Courses, with this self-study audio tape program. It is a good option for learning more about arthritis if a Self-Help Course isn't available in your area.

In Control

This program is another good option if a Self-Help Course isn't available in your area. Six lessons are presented on videotape and supplemented by a workbook and audio tapes.

Reliable Information at Your Fingertips

You know the adage: Knowledge is power. In addition to the classes and programs listed above, the Arthritis Foundation has information available in a variety of formats. With so many options for learning, you're sure to find just the information you need.

Information Hotline

The Arthritis Foundation is the expert on arthritis, and is only a phone call away. Call toll-free at 800/283-7800 for automated information on arthritis 24 hours a day. Trained volunteers and staff are also available at your local chapter to answer questions or send you a list of physicians in your area who specialize in arthritis.

Arthritis Foundation Web Site

If you're computer savvy and enjoy surfing the Internet, learn about arthritis 24 hours a day via the Arthritis Foundation's site on the World Wide Web. Check out http:// www.arthritis.org for information on programs and services, publications, local chapter activities and more.

Publications

A number of publications are available to educate you and your family about important issues such as medications, exercise, diet and other day-to-day considerations.

Booklets. You can learn about arthritis-related conditions, medications and caring for yourself with the more than 60 booklets and brochures published by the Arthritis Foundation. Single copies are available from your local chapter free of charge. Call your local chapter or 800/283-7800 for a listing of available booklets.

Arthritis Today. This award-winning bimonthly magazine gives you the latest information on research, new treatments and tips from experts and readers to help you manage your condition. Each issue also includes a variety of helpful articles to make your life with arthritis easier and more rewarding. A one-year subscription to Arthritis Today is yours free when you become a member of the Arthritis Foundation. Annual membership is $20 and helps fund research to find cures for arthritis. Call 800/933-0032 for membership and subscription information. Arthritis Today is also available nationwide on the newsstand, so look for it in your local bookstore.

Books. Self-care books are available from the Arthritis Foundation to help you learn more about your condition and how to manage it. Check your local bookstores, contact your local Arthritis Foundation chapter or call 800/207-8633 for available titles.

Audiovisual libraries

Many Arthritis Foundation chapters have audio and videotapes available for purchase or loan. Topics range from exercise to relaxation, and will vary from one chapter to another. Call your local chapter for a list of titles and prices.

Remember the Arthritis Foundation In Your Will

The mission of the Arthritis Foundation is to support arthritis research and to improve the quality of life for those affected by arthritis and related conditions. Planned giving is an important part of fulfilling this mission. The Foundation's planned giving department offers a wide variety of gift planning options, including estate gifts and gifts that provide donors with lifetime income.

We hope you decide to include a gift to the Arthritis Foundation in your will. Your greatest benefit from doing so will be the personal satisfaction of making a difference in the struggle against arthritis and related conditions. For more information on giving opportunities, call the Arthritis Foundation's planned giving department at 404/872-7100.

MORE GREAT BOOKS FROM THE ARTHRITIS FOUNDATION!

Beyond Chaos: One Man's Journey Alongside His Chronically Ill Wife
Discover how living with his wife's chronic illness brought a new level of trust and intimacy to author Gregg Piburn's marriage, and let his experiences guide you through your own journey.
346 pages
#835-214
$14.95

Health Organizer: A Personal Health-Care Record
Keep your medical and insurance records in one easy-to-find location, and track your symptoms with useful prompts in this spiral-bound, tabbed organizer.
144 pages
#835-207
$11.95

250 Tips for Making Life with Arthritis Easier
Packed with simple ideas for making daily tasks easier on your joints and less fatiguing, this book gives you ideas that you can start using today!
88 pages
#835-202
$9.95

Your Personal Guide to Living Well with Fibromyalgia
This hands-on workbook gives you the tools you need to take control over your condition and start down the path toward wellness.
224 pages
#835-203
$14.95

Toward Healthy Living: A Wellness Journal
This beautifully designed, spiral-bound journal contains inspirational quotes and pain and mood charts that help you track the progress of your health.
144 pages
#835-205
$9.95

The Arthritis Foundation's Guide to Alternative Therapies
This compendium of nearly 90 alternative therapies is a complete guide of the most-used unconventional therapies and the scientific research that supports or dispels any claims, myths or hype associated with them.
304 pages
#835-220
$24.95

PLACE YOUR ORDER TODAY!
1-800-207-8633

Operators are available to take your order
Monday – Friday, 8 a.m. – 5:30 p.m. EST

SOURCE CODE: CLPAGE

About the Author

Kathleen Lewis, RN, MS, LPC, CMP

Kathleen Lewis lives with many chronic illnesses on a daily basis: systemic lupus erythematosus, fibromyalgia, Sjögren's syndrome, Raynaud's phenomenon and osteo-arthritis. Through her writing, Kathleen shares the story of how she has learned to choose and celebrate life when faced with illness.

She is a registered nurse, a licensed professional counselor, a certified medical psychotherapist, a Stephen Minister, and has a Master of Science degree in rehabili-tative counseling with a specialty in chronic illness. Kathleen has worked extensively with developing, testing, training and teaching the Systemic Lupus Self Help course. She has been published extensively and speaks around the world to professional and patient groups.